I0134991

Resistance Workout

The Easiest Way to Strengthen Your Muscle

(Resistance Band Exercises for Strength Training and Mobility)

Eunice Kautzer

Published By **Jackson Denver**

Eunice Kautzer

All Rights Reserved

Resistance Workout: The Easiest Way to Strengthen Your Muscle (Resistance Band Exercises for Strength Training and Mobility)

ISBN   978-1-77485-909-4

All rights reserved. No part of this guidebook shall be reproduced in any form without permission in writing from the publisher except in the case of brief quotations embodied in critical articles or reviews.

Legal & Disclaimer

The information contained in this ebook is not designed to replace or take the place of any form of medicine or professional medical advice. The information in this ebook has been provided for educational & entertainment purposes only.

The information contained in this book has been compiled from sources deemed reliable, and it is accurate to the best of the Author's knowledge; however, the Author cannot guarantee its accuracy and validity and cannot be held liable for any errors or omissions. Changes are periodically made to this book. You must consult your doctor or get professional medical advice before using any of the suggested remedies, techniques, or information in this book.

Upon using the information contained in this book, you agree to hold harmless the Author from and against any damages, costs, and expenses, including any legal fees potentially resulting from the application of any of the information provided by this guide. This disclaimer applies to any damages or injury caused by the use and application, whether directly or indirectly, of any advice or information presented, whether for breach of contract, tort, negligence, personal injury, criminal intent, or under any other cause of action.

You agree to accept all risks of using the information presented inside this book. You need to consult a professional medical practitioner in order to ensure you are both able and healthy enough to participate in this program.

Table Of Contents

Chapter 1: The Fundamentals

We should begin by getting a better understanding of what resistance bands are.

The resistance band an elastic band with a light weight that can be used for strength training. It's a method of strengthening or stretching your muscles to improve fitness, physical therapy or for aesthetics. Bands of resistance cause muscular contraction. When you pull on the band, this contraction motion will help increase the strength of your muscles.

At first, these bands were initially used for rehabilitation for those suffering from injuries to their muscles or from sports. This is due in part to the fact elastic bands do not put the same pressure as weightsdo, making sure that joints as well as any other area of your body remain protected during your exercise. This means that you'll be able to gradually regain your loss of strength without stress.

Resistant bands differ based on the shape and size, handle color, and whether they are looped or not. looped.

Different kinds of resistance bands

Here are the principal kinds of resistance bands that are available:

Therapy band

Like the name suggests this, the use of the bands is commonplace in rehabilitation environments. Therapy band as being a smooth, thin elastic band that provides moderate resistance. They are comfortable for your body and do not have handles.

They are ideal to help you recover from your injury as you work the steps to gain stabilization and basic strength. Because they tend to be less heavy than other bands doctors may suggest exercising your muscles slowly using these bands after an injury. Therapy bands are also a great option to help with mental rehabilitation.

Bands of resistance that are compact

Compact resistance bands are similar to cord bands that have two handle (or clips) on either side - at times, they may include ankle or wrist cuffs. They're also referred to in the form of "fit tube" tubular or resistance bands.

They come in different shades and resistance levels, and generally longer than others (approximately 4 feet in length). They must also have an anchor system that can be attached to the door to provide support.

The Fit Tube bands are primarily employed to strengthen the arms, the lower part of the body along with the upper and lower body. Because of their numerous uses, they're ideal when you're looking for a versatile band to train at home.

Mini bands/fit loop bands

These are flat, tiny bands that form an unbroken loop of about 4 inches in length. It is a great exercise tool if your routine includes a lot of low-body, floor-based exercises.

Mini bands are ideal to strengthen your hips glutes and legs. They are a perfect fit for your thighs, ankles, knees, and calves while you exercise. Fit loops are ideal for lateral workouts that demand to keep your form. they can also make routine exercises like squats more difficult.

It's not uncommon for knees to collapse during squats, it is usually due to the glutes and abductors being weak. The use of these bands makes it possible to see if your knees are performing properly and to adjust your posture. If your exercise routine involves lots of squats you should consider purchasing the fit loop band.

Figure 8 Bands

These bands can be described as a tube with the form of figure 8 with handles made of plastic on both ends. With double handles, and being smaller by length (approximately 20 inches) makes them perfect to help build strength in the upper body especially around the arms.

The bands in Figure 8 are commonly used in a variety of functional exercises. They are also excellent for conditioning because they can isolate certain muscles during training. You can also incorporate them into Pilates and physical therapy.

Ring resistance bands

It is possible to describe this tube band as having multiple chain links, with handles at either end. They come with soft plastic handles.

With ring-resistant bands, it is simple to alter the size of the grip (thereby either loosening or tightening the resistance) regardless of the position you hold the band, you'll always have a hand. Based on your specific workout or grip you could make use of this band to exercise your feet, legs and stomach, hands, arms, neck and shoulders.

Lateral resistance bands

The band appears to be it's a long, wide band with Velcro cuffs on both sides even when not in use. It is common to wrap the cuffs around the ankles to exercise the lower body, particularly the hips, thighs, and glutes.

The the lateral resistance band is a favorite for lateral walks during strength training. It's a great method to warm up prior to starting more intense cardiovascular exercises which aids in enhancing the stability of your ankle and knee joint stability.

Bands to pull up

This is a specific type of resistance band that is designed for those who would like to do more reps, and who are unable to perform bodyweight pull-ups on their own.

The band allows you to pull-up without putting too much stress onto your arms. It's an ideal way to start your the upper body exercises.

With the aid of a pull-up bands, you can build your biceps, rhomboids trapezius and lats. The longer you use this piece of equipment, the more quickly your muscles begin to appear more defined, and soon you'll be able to perform pull-ups without assistance by the band.

To make sure you're benefiting the most from this band, it is important to use the right resistance. The heavier bands will are more resistant than the thinner ones. If you don't, you might be pushing yourself hard during your routine , but not getting the most benefit from your pull-ups. In addition to assisted pull-ups, these bands can also be a useful instrument for lower-body exercises.

Flat resistance band

Like the name suggests the band appears to be an ordinary band that is made from flattened material. The flat nature of this band makes it ideal for those who are undergoing physical therapy. The bands are great for anyone who wants to tone or tighten any muscle category. Some examples of exercises can be done with an elastic resistance band include standing hammer curls and standing high row. Other examples include lunges, lateral raises, and chest presses.

Please note: As you may have seen, therapy bands as well as flat bands do overlap in terms of their function and appearance.

Tube band

Tube-style resistance bands are generally circular, with handles at both ends. When you first glance at the band it may look like a small jump rope. They are great for pushing and pulling movements like a band overhead press. These are among the most flexible bands that are available. They function as a dumbbell, as well as a cable pulley.

Chapter 2: Benefits Of Resistance Bands

What are the chances that you will gain by using resistance bands into your workout routine?

Improves the effectiveness of exercise

Resistance bands training is an entirely different approach to exercise in comparison to weight training. Instead of lifting the weight they keep your muscles in constant tension, resulting in that you will notice a substantial increase in the performance of each and every exercise.

Furthermore, you could give your body different stimuli by discovering new ways to exercise that aid in its growth and adaptation.

Aids in focusing your attention

Resistance bands can make you stronger, even though it's more challenging than weight-lifting. It can help improve your body's overall fitness and functional strength. All it boils down to how you practice the frequency and intensity of your practice. you are working out. In the beginning, when you start using resistance bands, it may feel fragile, but after regular use and some time, you'll gain complete control.

Furthermore, you'll need an intense concentration to control the release of the band and the tension. Don't leave them to snap.

Works multiple muscles

Most exercises using resistance bands are compound, meaning they exercise multiple muscles at the same time. Compounded exercises burn more calories and require more energy, resulting in an all-body exercise. Additionally, because you must adjust to the changes in resistance bands and demands, you must have precise movements.

As I mentioned previously that using bands may be a little unsteady at first because of the constant tension. This means you'll have to focus on your core and work harder to maintain your posture and control. Based on the extent to which you stretch your band, your workouts will become more difficult and will increase your the physical strength and stability.

The stabilizing muscles are activated.

Doing your best to maintain form and control builds your core strength, and concentrates on stabilizing muscles at the same time. Resistance band exercises stimulate muscles that are that are known as stabilizers. Their purpose is to support the body and help stabilize it, therefore they are ideal to build stability and core strength.

Instrument for functional training

In comparison to conventional exercises, working out with resistance bands requires more. This is beneficial because it strengthens joints and permits more natural movements throughout your day routine.

If you can build such strength, it will help you achieve your fitness goals, and also helps you stay healthy and fit throughout your life.

Promotes better form

Sometimes, you may be performing some specific workout and you'll need to apply momentum to finish the last couple of reps. If you are using resistance bands it gets a lot more difficult.

Because you must maintain tension throughout the entire session Your muscles will be working all time and the result of each repetition is satisfied - not just when you finish your round. This helps your growth and growth, which makes elastic bands a great training device for building total body strength.

They teach you to recognize what's not working and what's going on.

Since you control how you use the band - the setting and movement, the angle, and even the position - you must be able to pay attention to the feeling of each exercise to be able to identify the parts you're working on.

When you're sure you're hitting the right muscles, you should concentrate on pushing them in the right way to the end in order to get an entire contraction. It will improve the effectiveness of your workouts if you utilize these bands in correctly.

They are light

If you'd like to work out at the comfort at home, without taking your space too much or simply don't have the time to go into the fitness center, it may benefit to have an assortment of resistance bands. It's also simple to take those sets to your gym. Simply put them into your gym bag and you're ready to go.

In addition, if you wish to make sure you are working out however you travel a lot then you could carry them around and use them anyplace. You can even take them with you on vacation to maintain your fitness during your vacation.

Who is the right person to use Resistance Bands?

Based on the information we've provided up to now, you can likely see that everyone can make use of resistance bands to meet fitness goals. Below are some groups that will get the most value from the bands:

Anyone looking to bulk up

If your goal is to increase strength and bulk then you can use dumbbells and machines for resistance bands to provide your muscles with a an exciting new stimulus to stimulate development. They can also be used in your barbell workouts to boost the intensity and strength of your neuromuscular system.

Are you looking to shed some weight?

The combination of strength training, cardio as well as a balanced diet can make losing weight simple. Use the bands as part of your routine of exercise However, make sure you use them in a full-body workout for the most effective outcomes.

For example, you can do back rows as well as squats and a chest press using the band for a full-body circuit. This will help burn calories and strengthens muscles and helps shed the extra weight in time.

Older adults

For people who are 60 or older, it could be quite challenging in their body to perform using the standard weights in the gym. The use of resistance bands can help to maintain strength and muscle mass without putting too much pressure on the body. Some medical professionals have advised against using that you use resistance bands to be the most method of stopping osteoporosis and enhancing bone strength.

Women who are pregnant

It is crucial to do an exercise routine during pregnancy to boost mood and energy levels, as well as quality of sleep and, perhaps most important getting ready for the birth of your child. But, it's not the right time to begin an intense weight-training program since it isn't secure.

High repetitions (15 up to 20) using resistance bands is fantastic for a little bit of strengthening your muscles and is completely secure. You can exercise every major muscle group with ease using just only one light and one medium band.

Chapter 3: What Are Resistant Bands Used For?

As mentioned previously, resistant bands serve two purposes:

* General fitness

* Physical therapy

There are many kinds of athletes and practitioners falling within the two broad categories which are further discussed below:

Resistance Bands for Fitness

They include:

Training in sports

Many athletes make use of resistance bands to build specific muscles required to increase the level of their sports. For example martial artists can utilize resistance bands to increase their grip strength and upper arm strength which makes it easier to keep grips and chokes.

In the off-season, skiers can build muscles around their calves and thighs using resistance bands, so that when the season gets underway they'll be able to ski through the snow at a perfect angle effortlessly.

Aesthetics

One of the most effective ways to shape your body is to use resistance bands since they're in a better position to focus on specific areas than weights and machines. Resistance bands are the best option if you desire to achieve a specific appearance - sculpted abs toned arms, etc.

Dance

Resistant bands can be beneficial for dancers to improve their balance and strengthen their knees, thighs and calves. Dancers, as well as ballerinas, are able to use the bands to do barre exercises that strengthen muscles in the legs, which is essential to the success of their dancing routine.

A rigorous fitness routine

Programs for intense fitness like P90x require the use of elastic bands into their exercise routines because of the effectiveness they have in preparing muscles, and also because they are color-coded to the intensity levels which makes evaluating them easy. Training participants can complete various exercises using various levels of color and witness significant and undeniable improvements.

Bands of Resistance for Physical Therapy

The uniqueness of resistance bands is what makes them popular in physical therapy.

If you are injured by an area of muscle, other muscles tend to begin growing around it in order to help compensate for the weakness. But, this natural process may backfire, as it's less likely for an injured muscle to recover to its strength to its fullest. Resistance bands help physical therapists ensure that the muscle in question is the one that is rebuilding strength and not the muscles around it.

Since they're color-coded this makes it easier for physical therapists and physical therapists choose the level of resistance for their patients in accordance with their injury. To prevent straining muscles injured, patients are able to start at a moderate level, and then progress according to how quickly the muscles heal.

How to Select Resistance Bands for Starting

When you purchase resistance bands, make sure you take two or more of the same levels to have another option in the event you discover that you purchased one that is either too difficult or difficult to use. If it becomes too easy to use one band, you could change it to another to make the workout more difficult.

Furthermore, you can also use lighter bands for smaller muscle groups , and heavier ones that are for bigger muscle groups in order to help you get more out of your workout.

If you are a novice in resistance band, you'll first need to be aware of the various levels of resistance to make sure you find the best band for you.

Understanding the different levels of resistance

The amount of force generated by bands during workouts is known as"resistance level. The different level of resistance in the band is typically identified by colour-coding. Resistance bands come in four main kinds of resistance:

* Light

* Medium

* Heavy

* Extra-heavy

Regular exercise improves overall body strength and muscular tone and gives you the opportunity to progress to higher resistance levels.

Bands of light resistance (Yellow)

This kind of band is suitable for seniors or beginners, users who require light resistance or those who have sustained an injury. Yellow bands provide resistance between 2.5 up to 3.5Kgs.

Middle resistance bands (Green)

Resistance bands made of green are a fantastic alternative for general strength training exercises. They are resistant to around 3.6 up to 5.5Kgs.

Similar to that of yellow's resistance bands medium bands are appropriate for those in the early phases of recovery, those who haven't worked for a long time, or novices.

Resistance bands of heavy weight (Blue)

With a resistance of around 6 kilos, these large resistance bands are great for those who exercise often. They are also great for improving your endurance.

Resistance bands that can withstand extra weight (Black)

This kind of band is generally reserved for the best and strong practitioners who require greater resistance. They offer a resistance that is greater than 13kgs.

Chapter 4: Simple Resistance Band Workouts

Anyone Can Do

We'll now concentrate on exercises with a resistance band that any person can perform:

Upper Body Exercise The Shoulders

They include:

It's not necessary to be too technical The most efficient method to build the muscles in your shoulders is to know the anatomy of your shoulders. By knowing this you'll be able to understand the purpose for every workout and which muscles you should focus on, which will help you build more of a connection between your muscles and your mind.

We will not be examining each muscle in the shoulder only the four main muscles:

1. Trapezius

2. Posterior deltoid

3. Lateral deltoid

4. Anterior deltoid

The anterior deltoid muscles is located at the point where the chest and shoulder muscles meet. The main function of this muscle is raising the arms to the upwards direction however, it is required for pushing in a vertical plane. It is also an important role in moving your arms backwards towards the midline.

However, the deltoid lateral is the middle segment of shoulder muscles. It functions against the anterior deltoid, which is responsible for moving your arm inwards. In simple terms the lateral deltoid's function is responsible for abduction, while the anterior one is responsible for the adduction. The lateral deltoid plays a crucial role in reaching out to grab something. If you've ever attempted to carry things that were heavy or heavy objects and experienced the heat of the weight over your shoulder, then you have activated this muscle.

The posterior deltoid is another which folds in the muscle fibers that surround the spine. Similar to the lateral deltoid it's also an integral component of reaching as well as other tasks such as throwing and dressing.

In addition, there are trapezius muscles, which are triangular in shape. They are situated at the side of the neck and shoulders. Their purpose is to support arm movement and also the range of motion as well as the movement of the head.

Lateral raise

Because shoulders are extremely fragile joints, it is essential to strengthen them in order to prevent injuries to the rotator cuff as well as frozen shoulders and much more. A lateral lift is a isolation movement that strengthens the shoulder's deltoid muscle, which aids in building stronger shoulders. For this exercise:

* Place the band of resistance under both of your feet, and then stand straight.

* Hold either end of the bracelet with both hands.

* While holding the band on the front of your hips. lift your hands straight up to the level of your shoulders. You can then stretch them back to your sides.

* Maintain the position for one second, and then reduce you arms gently.

* Perform 2-3 sets of 8-15 repetitions.

Separate

This exercise can be great to improve your mobility and strengthen your shoulders. Here's how you can do it:

* Make sure your feet are at a height that is as wide as your shoulders and bend your knees slightly.

* Hold the bands' middle portion as large and high as your shoulders by using both hands with your palms facing downwards.

* Pull the band out and then back in till you can feel your shoulders contract. Make sure that you keep your arms straight for the all the duration.

* Slowly return to your original position.

* Work the same motion for 8-10 reps

Forward raise

S

This workout is great for your front shoulders. It provides similar benefits to the lateral lift, however it further exercises the shoulder's anterior muscles such as that of anterior deltoid.

To do it:

* Set your feet the same height as your shoulders, and then stand on your band's middle part.

* Keep the handles by your sides, with your thumbs facing inward with your palms facing the back.

* Move your right arm forward until it reaches the height of your shoulders, without locking the shoulders.

Begin by gently lowering your arms until they are back to a comfortable level. Repeat for 8-12 reps before switching to the opposite arm.

Overhead press

Share your thoughts on

This exercise is typically utilized to strengthen the anterior deltoid muscle of the shoulder. Here's how to perform it:

As wide as your legs and feet large as your shoulders, place yourself over the middle portion of the tube band.

* Take both handles and stretch them upwards until your hands are shoulder height with your palms facing upwards, and your thumbs touching your shoulders.

* Pull on the bands upwards till you've fully extended your arms.

* Then slowly lower your arms towards the floor.

* Do 8 to 10 repetitions.

Reverse fly

This exercise is beneficial to those who perform exercises that require bending forward or sitting for the majority of the time since it can improve posture. It targets shoulders, upper arms and the upper back.

Here's how:

* Stand tall in the middle in your group.

* Take both ends, and connect them with your hands, so that it is crossed through your lower legs.

Bend your knees slightly forward as you pull your hips towards your back and make sure that your spine is in a neutral position and straight.

* TIP: Make sure your knees are bent slightly during the exercise.

* Pull the band upwards and outwards until your hands reach the level of your chest or go over.

* Bring your shoulder blades towards each other , in a contracting motion.

* Keep your position over a few seconds before slowly returning to the original position.

Overhead band pull-apart

This exercise helps improve posture, mobility and stability. It targets the shoulders tricepsmuscles, and the back.

Here's how to accomplish it:

* Grab the band with both hands, straight over your head.

• Gently lower your arms until the level of your shoulders while pulling away the band. Ensure that you are pressing your hands towards the sides.

Keep your posture for a few seconds before slowly returning to the original position.

* Be sure that your shoulders are kept to your ears when exercising.

Face pulls of the banded face

This exercise helps strengthen those muscles in the middle of trapezius as well as the rear deltoids, as well as rhomboids.

To do this exercise:

* Put your resistance band around a bar with a vertical angle to keep it at eye level.

* Grab the opposite end by placing either hand close to each other with palms facing downwards. You must tilt your torso to the side as well as keep the knees bent.

Then you can pull the band towards your face and separate your hands during the process. Make sure that your scapula is fully elongated while your arms are straight and out.

* Reposition the band gently back to its original position.

Shrugs with bands

This exercise is great to build the trapezius as well as the Rhomboid muscles. To do this exercise:

* Place your feet on the middle part of your band while keeping your feet separate by the shoulder length.

* Hold either looped end of your band with either hand while maintaining an upright and stable posture.

Now turn your shoulders up, retaining the up position for an additional second.

* Releasing your shoulders slowly towards the starting position.

* Repeat for 8-12 reps.

Retraction of the scapula.

Here's how you can complete this exercise:

Wrap your band around your wrists. Lift your arms to an angle that is right and your fingers pointed upwards , and your palms facing one another.

• Tighten your core prior to slowingly rotating your elbows to the side while squeezing your shoulder blades into. Make sure that your core stays tight and don't arch your back when you work.

* Press your shoulder blades for two seconds, then let them go and return your arms back to their original position. Complete 2-3 sets doing 10-15 reps.

External rotation of the shoulder

This exercise targets the same areas of the rowing exercise above. Here's how to perform it:

* To begin to sit straight, you must be sitting in the chair

* Hold the band in your hands with a little tension by either hand.

* Position your elbows at your sides bent at a right angle.

* Then slowly pull the band towards your side, making sure that your elbows remain close to your center.

* As you go through the motion you pinch your shoulder blades, just like you did during the row.

Release your band slowly, then return to the original position.

* Perform 2 sets of 8-15 reps.

Chapter 5: Chest Workouts

In the majority of exercises the chest is usually the muscle group that is most neglected. There are four main muscles: back, legs, abdominals and chest.

A weak chest muscle puts unneeded stress on your other muscle groups, which makes vulnerable to injuries in your daily activities and workouts.

The muscles that are the primary ones in the chest are:

* Serratus anterior

* Pectoralis minor

* Pectoralis major

Pectoralis major originates at the sternum (breast bone) and is inserted into the lower half of your collar bone. The muscle's fibers extend outside of the humerus (upper arm bone). The pectoralis's functions major are to move your arms upwards, and then directing your arms upwards from your side across your body.

Pectoralis minor runs from the front portion of the shoulder blades up to the third and fifth ribs. The pectoralis minor muscle supports your shoulder blades to the rib cage in pressing motions.

Serratus anterior, also known as a fan shape muscle that runs from the 1st through 8th ribs. It folds into the shoulder blade's within the boundary. Similar to the pectoralis minor muscle and pectoralis major, it uses the rib cage to support your shoulders during press-ups, for example, as well as the bench press.

The chest muscles that are the primary ones are in sync with the triceps and biceps as well as the and deltoid, to move your arm with press and chest fly exercises.

Below are some simple chest exercises:

Chest press

To begin to begin, stand or sit

* Get your resistance band, and secure it to your back, at the top of your chest.

* Grab either handle of the band with both hands.

Start with bending the elbows while place your hands in front of your chest.

Relax your arms to straighten them completely in front of you.

* Slowly return back to the original position.

* Perform 2-3 Sets of between 8 and 15 repetitions.

Pullover that is lying

* Take the tube band and secure it in a low place

* Lay down on the floor, with your head facing toward the anchor. Hold the end of the band in both hands.

* Lift your arms to the left hand over your head. Then make them stretch by stretching them forward to the left of your anchor.

* Gently bend your elbows to cross your torso until the handles are on the knees' side.

* Remain in the position you were in earlier.

* Repeat for 8-10 reps.

Incline chest press

To do it:

* Attach the middle part of the band with an anchor on the slope seat.

Sit in a comfortable and hold one of the handles in each hand, and then raise the band until it is at your shoulder at a level.

Apply your bandage until you've all the way extended to the chest.

* Slowly lower your arms to their starting position.

* Do 10-12 reps

Bench press

Share with Pi

To do it:

* With your back pressed against the bench, and the tube band secured underneath the bench, grasp the handles using your hands.

* Position your hands on the shoulder so that your thumbs are touching your shoulders front.

* Straighten your arms around your chest until they are fully extended. When you are at the top, you can move your hands in a direction towards each other.

* Slowly return your arms back to their original position.

* Do 10-12 times.

Band of resistance

This exercise focuses on the pectorals.

Here's how:

The band should be wrapped around a solid horizontal fencing post, bar or pole.

* Hold both ends of your handles or band while facing your back towards the pole.

* With a more wide posture (one foot ahead one of the others) place your arms sideways in a straight line to your chest.

* Move your arms towards the side of your body, with an incline in your elbows.

* Return your arms to their starting position for 3 seconds.

* Repeat for 8-12 reps.

Make sure your elbows are not above the shoulders when you workout.

Low crossover with wide-stance

This exercise stretches the muscles of the chest.

Here's how:

The band should be placed under your feet. Then, increase your legs beyond shoulder width. The wider the legs you spread out the more you will work your chest.

* Keep the handles to the sides of your hips.

* As your core muscles are tightened by pulling one hand upwards and then place it in front of your body until you're near your shoulder while maintaining an incline in your elbow.

* Stay in the position for one second

* Repeat this using the opposite arm, and then keep switching sides.

* Repeat for 8-12 reps.

One arm fly with crossover that has band

* Tie the band below your knee, or walk onto your knee, leaving the remainder of it on the opposite side of your body.

* Grab the band with the palm on the side that is secured, maintaining an unnatural bend at the elbow.

* Beginning with a little bit more tension in the band pull it towards the front over to the shoulder on the opposite side.

* Hold this position for one second before slowly returning to the starting position.

* Do 8-10 reps for each side, until you've completed one set.

Fencer crossover pull

Attach the band to an upright pole just above your knee.

* While standing with the band to the body's side grasp it with your opposite hand, so that it crosses your body.

* With a slight bend of your elbow take the band off the opposite hip by pulling it up front of you , and across your body to shoulder height - similar to the way you would pull a sword out of its sheath.

* Extend your elbow upwards away from your body as you pull your hand away and up above.

Reduce your arm slowly, gently bent your elbow when you return to the starting position.

* Do 8-10 reps each side for a complete set.

Decline chest press

This workout targets on the chest's lower muscles, which help create a bigger and stronger chest.

Here's how:

* Wrap the strap around the upper part of your back, securing it with traps, and then grasp the ends.

Place your hands on the sides of your chest.

* Place one foot on top of the other foot to create more impact.

* While your elbows are bent slightly, spread your hands outwards to the side.

* Stay in this position for while prior to returning back to your original position.

8. Repeat for 8-12 repetitions.

Inline press variation

This exercise increases the power of your muscles as well as strengthens your upper pectoral muscles.

Here's how:

* Attach the band in a place that is higher that your head.

* Hold either of the handles of the band with each hand, with the front facing you.

Step in the direction of your body to create a small tension in your.

* Put one foot on top of the other to ensure stability and to bring your back to the correct position.

Now, with an incline in your elbows, move your arms up towards your body, pointing downwards to the point that your arms are almost touching.

* Slowly bring your arms back until you hold the shoulder blades and then extend your chest.

* Repeat this motion 10-12 times.

Chapter 6: Back Exercises

If you've ever felt back pain, you are aware of how painful and uncomfortable it can be.

A majority of 60-80 percent of adults suffer from lower back discomfort. Because your back is involved in nearly every movement performed by your body and can cause pain, it could affect your everyday activities. Training your back muscles can improve your motion range and helps to prevent or treat nonspecific back pain.

These are the main muscles of the back:

* Erector Spinae The muscle that runs through the spine.

* Trapezius (traps) * Trapezius (traps) previously mentioned these muscles start at the neck's back and stretch all up to the mid-back.

* Rhomboids These muscles are located found in the middle part of your back.

* Latissimus dorse (lats) These muscles extend from the area under your armpits to the side that runs along your back.

Row to the right

This exercise is perfect to target your traps.

To do it:

Place your feet on the middle portion of the band, shoulder length.

* Hold the handles of the band by your palms, and pull them until you stand tall. Place them in side of your thighs.

* Bring your band up to your shoulders by using your elbows. Make sure your elbows are bent, forming the shape of a high V.

* Slowly lower your arms to the original position.

* Row to 10-12 times.

The row

This exercise is great to correct posture and strengthen the upper back.

To do it:

* Sit on your knees with your legs extended to the side with a slight bend between your knees.

The band should be placed beneath each foot, then hold the handles in either hand.

* Begin with tension in your band, and bend your elbows to a right angle.

* Gently pull the band in your direction while you extend your elbows out beyond your body by gently pressing your shoulder blades while you go about this.

* Do 3 groups of between 8 and 15 repetitions.

Lat pulldown

This exercise is designed to strengthen the upper back. Here's how you can do it:

* Wrap the band over a horizontal bar or to the branch of a strong tree to secure it.

* Kneel in front of the anchor until you've got the band right in front of you.

If you have your arms spread over your head, and your hands slightly larger than shoulder width grasp either side from the elastic band.

While you squeeze your back muscles your back, pull the band towards the floor while keeping the elbows bent.

* Lift your hands until they are at the level of your shoulders, and after which you gently bring them back to their starting position.

* Perform 10-12 reps.

Standing Ys

This short, easy workout will strengthen your back muscles in the upper part of your body. Here's how:

• Stand tall and have your feet about the same size of your shoulders.

* Wrap the miniband in either hand , and then extend your arms to the side of your head.

* The band should be pulled apart, keeping your core muscles engaged, and use your back muscles in the upper part of your body to resist the force.

* Release slowly and return to your starting position.

* Repeat for 10-12 reps.

Deadlift with banded bands

* Wrap either end of the band around both feet, then stand tall in a wider-then-your-shoulder-width stance.

* Squat down and grip the band with your hands at the center.

With your butt protruding as well as your lower back arched slightly, you can pull upwards this band till your spine is straight.

* Repeat for 8-10 reps.

Start by using a band that is light and ensure that your back is not bent forward as you work out to prevent injuries.

Stiff-legged deadlift

This exercise targets the lower back and hamstrings if executed properly. To do it:

* Stand at the mid-section of your band. Then do a squat to grasp two ends using your hands.

Maintain the upper part of your back straight in an upright, natural posture and lower back arched slightly.

• Pull the elastic band upwards until you stand upright.

The band Banded Good Mornings

For this exercise:

If you have your feet wider than your hips and the resistance band underneath both feet.

Hold the handles in your hands and raise your hands and secure your band where your shoulders and neck meet. Tension should be taken care of by your body, not by the arms.

* While your abs and glutes are contracted, pull your hips forward while dropping your the torso. The majority of your movements should be performed around your hip joints and your knees must be bent slightly. There should be no motion in your spine.

* When your torso has become close to your floor maintain the position for two seconds. You'll feel some force on the rear of your legs.

If you have a spine that is neutral move your hips forward, then stretch your glutes back to your original posture.

* Repeat for 10-12 reps.

Lat pulses with bands

Place your feet in the ground or on a on a yoga mat with your head towards the ceiling and your ankles underneath your hips. Make sure that your whole body starting from the head and ending at your toe is in a straight position.

• Lift your head a bit off the floor However, keep your head in a downward direction to avoid stressing your shoulders or your neck.

* Grab all ends with your hands. Your elbows should point toward the back with your arms straight with your palms up.

Lift your arms gently off the floor to engage your back muscles. Keep the posture of your arms towards your sides throughout the entire move. Don't be worried if the range of motion isn't that great since this move isn't that easy. Just go wherever you want to.

* Slowly return to your original position and repeat the exercise for 8-10 reps.

Banded Bird Dog

* Stand on all fours, placing your hands beneath your shoulders, knees beneath hips, with your toes tied.

* Wrap the band around one foot while the other is wrapped around the hand.

After your hips and torso are in a good position then stretch the other arm and leg. While stretching the leg, ensure that the motion is solely through the extension of your hip. your leg should be aligned with your torso. You must not bend your back. There must not be any tension of the spinal erectors.

If you move beyond your head, will feel the traps below acting in a reflexive manner.

* When the leg and arm are fully stretched, exhale.

Return your leg arm back to its original position.

* Repeat for 10-12 reps.

Bent over rows

Do this:

* Standing with your legs shoulder-width apart put the resistance band underneath your feet while keeping your feet slightly pointing out.

Keep your back straight with your chest elevated, the core tight and knees bent slightly and then bring your hips forward.

If you are able to keep your elbows extended then pull the band toward your chest, squeezing your shoulder blades and bringing them to the back.

* Stay in the position for two seconds before slowly releasing before returning to the original position.

* Repeat for 10-12 reps.

Chapter 7: Arm Workouts

The muscles in your arms are diverse which work "hand in hand'-no meaning intended -to enable your body to carry out various actions and tasks.

Before we dive into the various muscles it is vital to understand the four major kinds of motions that are associated by your arms.

* Adduction is the motion of a portion of the body towards the core, such as moving your arms to the side and resting on your torso.

* Abduction It is the movement of a part that is a part of your body to the side as in raising your arms outwards and away from your torso.

The Flex movement will bring two body parts closer to one another, similar to your forearm and upper arm.

* Extension: This movement will increase the distance between two parts of the body like the elbow being stretched straight.

The muscles of the upper arm muscles are divided into two parts:

* The posterior part of the compartment

* The posterior compartment

Anterior Compartment

This area is situated the front of the main bone of the upper arm the humerus. The muscles that make up this area comprise:

* Biceps brachii This muscle is usually known as the Biceps. The biceps are a pair of heads, which start from the front and back of your shoulders. They join to join around your elbows. The role of the biceps is assist with flexion and adduction of the upper arm.

* Brachialis: The muscle is located beneath the biceps. It acts in a way of bridging muscles of the ulna and the humerus. It is crucial to flex the forearm.

* Coracobrachialis located close to at the shoulders, the muscle permits the shoulder to bend as well as the adduction and extension of the upper arm. It also aids for stabilizing the humerus of the shoulder joint.

Posterior compartment

This is located behind the humerus, and contains the two muscles that follow:

* Triceps brachii running along the humerus This muscle is usually known as the triceps. The triceps assist in the stretching and flexion of your forearm as well as stabilizing the shoulder joint.

* Anconeus triangular muscle is small and sometimes thought of as being an extension for the triceps. It's responsible for rotating the forearm and stretching your elbow.

Below are some simple resistance band exercises that can be done on the arm:

Seated Biceps Curl using a resistance band

This workout targets both triceps as well as the biceps. Here's how to perform it:

* With your feet spread Sit on a bench, stool or chair.

* Place on one side of the band beneath your left foot. Hold the other end with your right hand.

* By leaning forward slightly and putting the elbow of your hand that is banded upon your

right leg. You can place your left hand on your left thigh, or put them on the side.

Maintain your back aligned and keep your core muscles engaged.

Begin by placing your arms at a right angle making the band tight.

* Now , move your right hand towards the shoulder. Keeping your shoulders in place, and focus on pulling your hands towards your bicep.

* Perform 10 to 12 repetitions for each arm.

Band Triceps Kickback

This exercise basically sculpts the triceps muscles and stimulates the core up to a certain level. Here's how you can do it:

* Place your feet on at the same width as your hips. Then, place the band under your feet.

* Hold either handle in your hands with your palms facing towards the inside.

With your core stretched, your back straightened and your knees bent slightly to the side, bend your knees slightly forward at your waist. Pull your arms towards an angle of right.

With your elbows tied to your sides, extend your arms upwards while keeping your arms further behind. Once you've reached the top, you can squeeze the band slightly.

Gradually lower your arms to their original position.

* Repeat for 15 reps.

Band curls to press

This exercise is excellent to build biceps and shoulders. It also works the core muscles while you brace to keep your balance. Here's how you can do it:

* Stand tall in the middle within your ensemble.

• Use an underhand grip for gripping the handles.

* While your chest is out and your core contracted, bring your hands towards your shoulders. Keep the elbows straight towards your sides.

* Once you've reached the shoulders, you can turn your wrists with your palms facing towards the forward direction.

* Push your head over until your arms fully stretch.

• Gently lower your hands down to your shoulders, flip them back to your palms, then return to your original posture.

* Do 15 reps.

Single-Arm Band Triceps Extension

This exercise strengthens and shapes the triceps and gives you strong, muscular arms. Place your arms close to the ears and hold your body still to the muscles of the triceps. Here's how to perform it:

* Stand tall and place your left hand slightly the direction of your right foot.

* Wrap the part of the band on your right foot, then grab the other with your right hand.

Reach your arm out over your head.

* With your arm in front of your ear and your core tightened bend your elbow until you bring the band down below your head.

• Straighten your arms above your head. pressing your triceps while doing it.

* Perform 15 reps for both arms.

Bow with Bands and Arrow

This workout is perfect for the shoulders, triceps and chest. Here's how you can accomplish it:

* Make sure you are standing with your core in place and your feet approximately the same width as your hips.

* Hold the ends of the band with either hand.

* Place your hands at the chest level

* Move your left arm toward the left side and keep your right arm within the chest. (Your right arm shouldn't extend past the mid-section in your physique).

You can adjust the tension of the band to make it enough to reach your starting point.

* Move your left arm to your left hand (away towards the left arm) similar to pulling an arrow in bow. Make sure your elbow is raised and pointed upwards.

* Slowly return to your original position.

Do 12-15 reps on each arm.

Resistance band pull-out

This workout is designed to strengthen the back, biceps and shoulders.

Here's how you can accomplish it:

* Keep your posture up with your core tight and your feet in a slack.

* Wrap the band over your body, hold each end with one hand.

* Make a right-angle at your elbows, by bending them, then extend this band over your lower back.

* As you are in this position, strengthen the back muscles by pressing your shoulder blades in a tense manner and ensuring that your shoulders

are closed as you open your arms in front of your body.

Then slowly bring your arms back to their original position in which your elbows are bent to an angle of right.

Banded Cuff Pivot

This exercise is perfect to strengthen the rotator cuffs and shoulders. To do it:

* Keep both feet joined.

* Hold the opposite one of the ends of the band in either hand. It is possible to alter the tension of the band simply by wrapping it around your hands several times until it's small enough.

* With your elbows pointed out , and your knees slightly bent to bring your hands beneath your chest - around the same distance as the bottom of your ribcage.

* With your right hand firmly attached to your body and your left hand pulled back from the sides and towards the left side, allowing your

elbow to rotate toward your waist. Feel the rotational force across your shoulders.

* Slowly return to your starting point.

* Do 12-15 reps for each arm.

Single-arm bent-over row

Here's how:

* Place one foot behind the other. Slightly lean forward, and then secure the band beneath the foot to the left.

* Place the other hand on your thigh to provide stability and support.

* Grab the handle using your other hand, keeping your palm facing outwards.

Spread your hand out to ensure that the band isn't loose.

* While keeping your elbow on your side draw your arm up until your elbow and shoulder are in line with each other.

* Keep the position for two seconds, then release gently then returning back to your original position.

* Repeat for 10-12 reps.

Keep your head up and your back straight.

Plank row

* Make sure you are in the position of high plank by looping an end over your right palm , and then holding the other with the left palm of your hand.

* Make tension on the band by slightly raising your right hand.

Keep your hips in their place and your core in place and your core engaged, pull your left elbow towards the hip's side.

• Slowly bring your arms to the position it was in before you complete one repetition.

* Perform 12-15 reps with each arm.

Plank taps

The band tied over your wrists take your high-plank posture.

Keep the core in place, bring your left hand two inches forward and then press the floor.

Return to your starting point and repeat using your right hand until you have completed 1 repetition.

* Perform 8-10 reps.

Chapter 8: Workouts For Core

The core muscles are located in the 'trunk' area of your body, which is the abdomen. The abdominal muscles control strength and are vital for stability, back health and general strength.

The core contains 35 muscle groups which comprise major and minor muscles. Here are the main muscles groups that make up your core:

* Rectus abdominis * Rectus abdominis: The rectus abdominis consists of the abdominal muscles that are located in the front commonly known as'six-pack abdominals.. This muscle group is responsible for your ability to bend and crunch and also helps to keep your core steady while doing push-ups or planks.

* Transverse abdominis: This muscle begins from the back of the rectus abdominis and runs across your body, ending below your rib cage, which is located on the lower side of your spine. The transverse abdominis performs an important role in protecting and helping support the spine.

* Obliques This muscle group includes two kinds of classification including the internal and the

63

external Obliques. They offer durability and support to the sides and front of the core. They are located on opposite sides of rectus abdominis, which is located on the front of the body. The obliques offer assistance when you are turning your torso around or bending towards the side.

* Erector Spinae This muscle group extends through the cervical region of the neck and into the lumbar area around the back's lower part. The erector spine is a one of the extensors of back. It is involved in movements like squatting, lifting or squatting. These muscles are vital to keep your core active and supplying stability and support to your spine.

* Multifidus: It is a muscle group situated on either side of your spine. They extend from your neck to the bottom of your pelvis. It plays a role in the stability and support of all vertebrae specifically in the lower lumbar region. The multifidus is usually connected to pain in your lower back.

Here are a few basic workouts using a band for resistance:

Banded Russian twist

* Place your legs in a straight line and keep them together.

* Wrap your band's middle to your feet. Grab the ends with both hands.

* While your heels are set to the floor, bend your knees, then pull either end of the band in by securing your hands.

Maintaining the back straight, and keeping your abdominal muscles tight by stretching your arms to the level of your eyes in front of your body. Lean to the side 45 degrees. Make sure that the band stays taut all the time you're doing your workout.

* Turn your lower body until you are to your right and then to the left side for one rep.

* Perform three sets with 12-15 repetitions.

Knee Pull

* With the middle section of the band wrapped around your left foot and the end of the band wrapped in both hands, start with the push-up

position (arms straight and balanced on your palms and toes).

* Once your core is tight throughout you, pull your left knee towards your chest, and then lower your head to join the knee.

• Stretch your leg using the left heel. Slowly return to your starting position, the push-up position.

Do 12-15 reps until you have completed 3 sets for each leg.

Elastic Teaser

* Wrap the band around the feet's soles. Then grasp each end with either hand.

With your legs in a row lay down on the floor, with your back facing up.

Place your arms at your sides.

* Move your body into V-position and pull the band using each arm.

Maintain the V-sit posture for 3-5 seconds before gradually lowering your body back to back to the beginning position.

* Do three sets, each of which is 12-15 repetitions.

Torso twist

With your feet separated in a hip-width direction Wrap the mid-section of the band underneath your feet. Then, grab the ends with either hand.

* Bend your elbows and raise your hands up to the height that your shoulders. Keep your palms straight ahead.

• With feet securely held in place, and knees bent slightly, turn your upper body until you are on your right.

* Slowly return to the center position, then move to the left side. It's 1 rep.

* Perform for 3 sets with 12-15 repetitions.

Bicycle crunch

* Wrap the band between your toes, move into a sitting position. Place your feet on the floor, and bend to the knees.

* With your fingertips gently over the inside of your ears Bend backwards to 45-degrees until your core muscles are engaged.

* Utilizing your core muscles to twist your torso, then bring your left elbow towards your right knee while you straighten your left leg.

Then, turn your waist so that you bring your right elbow closer to the left knee while you straighten your right leg. This is a complete repetition.

* Continue alternating your limbs for 12-15 reps.

Standing knee Tuck

Here's how:

Standing tall with your feet shoulder-width apart. then place the band in the soles of your feet in the middle.

* Lift your right knee toward the chest, while bringing your left elbow toward your right knee. Try putting your elbow on your knee, but not circling the shoulders.

Keep your balance, slowly return to the original position.

Switch to the opposite side, and repeat the process.

* Repeat on alternate sides for 10-12 reps.

Hollow body roll

* Lay on your back and wrap the wristband around your shoulders and arms extended straight across your head.

* Take the position of a hollow hold by swaying your shoulders and legs off the ground.

* Keep your biceps close to your ears, and your arms extended, move your entire body towards the left by using your core.

Once you're back on your feet (the starting position) then roll back to the left side and complete one rep.

* Repeat for 12-15 reps.

Dead bug with banded bands

For a full-on assault on the core muscles, make sure that you don't arch your back. Also, keep a neutral, stable position in your spine. This is how you can do it:

* Lay on your back, and then extend your legs.

The band should be looped through your foot on the right side, then grasp the other end with your left arm.

In order to maintain stability on the shoulder and the left arm then move your leg to straight in front of you.

* * If you're ready to it, raise your right hand to increase the intensity.

* When you stretch on your left leg you need to tighten your core. As you keep your movement under control then gently return to the beginning position.

* Do 10 repetitions each side. Do two sets.

Vertical scissors

* Sit on your back and keep the band looped around your ankles, and keep keeping your legs in a straight position.

Utilizing your arms to stabilize your body and your legs elevated from the floor at a 45-degree angle.

* While keeping your core in place and your core engaged, move your right leg up to keep the foot in line with your torso.

* Once you have returned your right leg back to the start position, raise the left leg up simultaneously and in a manner similar to the use of scissors which is why the name this exercise.

* The movement should have a rhythm and control, rather than erratic and unpredictable.

* Make sure you maintain your arms at all times during the move.

Chapter 9: The Glutes

"Glutes" are a very popular term used to describe the three types of gluteal muscles which originate from the pelvis and then fold into the femur. The word "glutus" is the Latin word meaning "gluotos," the Greek word that means "butt." These gluteal muscles are useful for jumping, sitting and running, walking and also for rotating hip joints. The three gluteal muscles that are the most important comprise:

* Gluteus maximus

* Gluteus medius

* Gluteus minimus

Gluteus minimus

Three gluteal muscles this is the most deep and the tiniest muscle group. The primary function of the gluteus maximus is to stabilize your pelvis/hips and abduct the thigh when doing activities like walking or sitting on one foot or running. In addition, its posterior part allows the external rotation of your thigh and its anterior section assists by allowing the internal rotation of your thigh.

Gluteus medius

Like its name implies the name, this muscle group is the gluteal muscles of the middle size that is located between the gluteus maximus and the gluteus minimus. The gluteus medius muscle is essential for movements like the medial, lateral and lateral rotation as well as hip abduction.

Furthermore, it plays a role in maintaining the stabilization of the pelvis which aids the gluteus minimus keep your pelvis aligned correctly during single-leg balance and moving.

Gluteus maximus

This is the strongest and largest gluteal muscle. It is among the strongest muscles that collaborates with other gluteal muscles to aid in hip rotation and to stabilize the pelvis. Furthermore the gluteus maximus plays a role in abduction, lateral rotation of the hips as well as hip extension, which permits the leg to extend backwards.

Below are some simple glute exercises that you can perform using your resistance band:

Bridge with Banded Glute

• Lie back on your back, with the knees bent, and the band looped just above your knees. With your feet a distance that your hips are, place your hands on your sides with your fingers nearly reaching the back of your heels.

* Firm your core and the lower back of your body against the floor.

* By pressing your feet on the floor, extend your hips until they are in line with your knees.

* Once you have reached the top, tighten your glutes.

* Slowly lower your hips slowly to return to your original position.

Clamshell with banded edges

* Lay on your left side and align your knees, ankles and hips.

* Loop the band over your knees. Then bend your knees at an angle of right.

* With your feet firmly together with your back straight and your core firmly engaged and your core engaged, lift your left knee and then open it.

• Gently lower your left knee until it is in line with the right knee. Make sure not to tilt back or lean forward.

* Perform 12-15 reps for each side.

Donkey kicks

* Loop the band just over your knees. Get on your feet with your hips aligned with your knees, and your shoulders are directly above your wrists.

Utilizing your core muscles to support your body, stretch your glutes and engage them by flexing your left leg, then kicking your foot up towards the ceiling.

Do not arch your back as you lift your foot up and try to keep your legs at a proper angle with your hips. shouldn't open your hips to the left when you raise your leg.

Then slowly lower the knee down to the floor to return to the original posture.

* Perform 12-15 reps per side.

Fire water source

* Loop the band over your knees.

You should stand on four legs, with your hips just above your knees, and your wrists and shoulders are aligned.

With your back straight with your abdominal muscles engaged in order to support the rest of your body, lift your left knee towards the left side.

* Bring your knee back to its original position.

* Perform 12-15 repetitions on your left side before changing to the other side.

Lifting the leg with a banded lie

Bandage your ankles.

* Lie in the side plank posture with your hips forward facing and your legs straight and your shoulder just over your elbow.

* While your spine is in a neutral place and your core firmly engaged to lift your leg the top straight up.

Be careful not to point your toes towards the sky after you've removed your leg. You may also pull your glutes into your thighs when you get to the top.

Then slowly return the leg back to the original position.

Leaning back too much from your hips and the toes pointed upwards work the quads instead of activating your glutes.

The banded marching Glute Bridge

The band should be placed at the level of your knees.

• Lie back lying on the back, and then bend your knees so that you be able to keep your butt, feet and shoulders placed onto the floor underneath your body.

* By bringing your heels to the floor then press your hips upwards.

* While your hips are elevated then slowly move one leg upwards in order to create an arc that runs diagonally from your shoulder and your chest and your knee towards your heel.

* Slowly lower the extended leg. Alternate to the opposite leg, completing 1 repetition.

* Perform 10-12 reps.

Kneeling leg lift

* Tie the band over your knees, then kneel.

Place one hand to the ground and the left hand behind your head. Alternatively, you can rest your head on your opposite knee.

* With your toes on the left foot, and your toes pressed down, extend your left leg over to the left side, allowing it to bring your hip in line to your leg. You can do this as far as you are able to extend your leg.

* To hold your band secure when working out place it under your right knee.

• Lower your leg in a controlled manner until your toes touch the floor. This will be 1 rep.

* Perform 10 to 12 repetitions of the left before switching to the right side.

Planks to support

* Imagine the plank posture with the band wrapped around the arches of your feet.

* Step forward using your left hand until your knee is directly below your hips , and just a couple of inches above the ground.

* Continue to follow with your right foot, and keep this position for at least a few seconds before returning to your starting position. This is one repetition.

Do 10-12 repetitions.

Kneeling and kicking butt kickback

* Get on your feet and stand up Wrap this band over your left arm, and beneath the arch of your left foot.

* While keeping the band straight and keeping your core brace in place, extend your left foot to the side.

Return to position from which you started.

* Do 10-12 reps per leg.

Kickbacks from the standing glute

* Standing tall, with your back in neutral, your with your core engaged and your hands on your hips.

* While your right leg is securely fixed Bend your knee slightly. (This is the leg that anchors).

While keeping either leg straight by squeezing your glutes until you can move your left leg behind you.

* Push as far as your fitness allows without leaning too excessively.

• Lower back to your left foot until it's in line with the right but do not allow it to come into contact with floor below.

Repeat the exercise with a slow speed.

* Perform 12-15 reps for each leg.

Chapter 10: The Lower Body Workout

Lower body exercises include:

Hips and Thighs

The muscles in the thigh are responsible for maintaining your balance. They permit rotation through the hips and legs, and keep your legs and hips in the proper alignment.

The most important thigh muscles comprise:

* Adductors They are located in the inner thigh, and extend from the pelvis up to the bones of the thigh (femur).

* Hamstrings: The muscles of the hamstring are located behind your thighs, being able to run from the hips, and then being folded into knees.

The quadriceps (quads) The quadriceps originates from the pelvis and femur and stretch all the way up to the hin bone (tibia) and the patella (knee cap).

Below are a few simple resistance band exercises for strengthening your the thighs and hips:

Standing hip Adduction

* Then, loop the other end of the band around an upright bar, and wrap the other end around your right ankle.

• Stand on your left leg closest towards the bar.

* Move your right leg front of you, and then over to your left leg then slowly return back to your starting place.

Make sure to keep your body upright.

Repeat 12-15 reps, and then move to the next leg.

* Work your core to keep your leg moving and stop your body from rotating or moving.

Two-leg side raise

* Lay down on your back, with your head resting on an arm that is extended or supported by your elbow for assistance.

* Lift the top leg towards the ceiling, making sure it is straight as you can.

* While your leg is suspending in air raise your second leg until it is parallel to it.

When your legs come into contact, lower the lower leg to the ground while the top leg stays suspended in the air.

* When your bottom foot is at the level of the floor, raise it again to align with the upper leg.

* Perform 10-12 reps prior to switching to the other side.

Your level of fitness will determine the size of your suspended leg. The higher up you set your foot, the more difficult it is to maintain it in suspension and the reverse is true.

Seated hip abduction banded with a banded

* Sit on a table or chair and place your feet down on the floor below the surface you.

* Wrap the band just above your knees , and wrap it around your legs.

While keeping your body straight, with the back upright and your chest lifted then push your knees outwards.

* Slowly bring your legs back to the starting position.

* Repeat for 10-12 reps.

During the move your feet may slide over their outside edges but make sure they stay in the same spot.

Side-to-side steps

Stand high with your feet at a shoulder width apart, with the band placed just above your knees.

* By pushing your butt forward while keeping your chest elevated and your knees bent slightly to form a half-squat.

Make sure you keep tension on the band throughout the exercise, make small steps to the left side while staying in the half-squat posture.

* Take 10-12 steps to the left side before moving to the right side.

* Standing side abduction of the hip

* Sit with your feet in a row and place the band just below your knees.

* Bend slightly and pull your hips back.

Maintaining a bent in your knee while maintaining your hips in the same direction by lifting one leg to your side. Do as much as your fitness level permits.

* Perform 8-10 reps for each leg.

Chair squats with banded legs

* With your legs at shoulder width apart, place the band above your knees. Then sit down in a chair.

* Intensify your band by pressing your knees to the outside, and then squatting to the point that your body touches the chair.

* Slowly increase the intensity and do 12-15 repetitions.

It is important to limit the time in close proximity to the chair.

Walk with Banded

* Make sure your feet are at the same height as your hips. Wrap this band over your ankles.

Maintain your glutes in a tight position and your core strong, pivot your hips forward and bend your knees slightly.

* Take one step forward, for 1 rep.

* Do 10 steps forward and 10 steps backwards in order to complete the set.

Keep your shoulders back with your spine straight.

Squat for the lateral leg lift

* While your feet are spread at a shoulder width apart Wrap this band over your legs just above your knees.

Place your hands either on your hips, or on your chest.

* Retract your hips as you bend your knees in order to lower your body to an squat.

Stand slowly then move your left leg to the left, while keeping your knee straight.

Then lower your leg toward the floor.

* Repetition the squat, and when you are again, lift your right leg to the left, making sure that you should keep the knee in a straight position.

Then lower the left leg to the floor , then do a squat for a second time to complete 1 full repetition.

* Repeat for 10-12 reps.

Make sure you keep your chest straight and your core engaged. Don't slouch or round your back.

Pulse of the hip bridge

The band should be wrapped around both of your thighs at the top of your knees.

* Lay on your back, with the knees bent with your your hands at your sides and your legs hip-width apart lying flat on the floor The your glutes are in a bridge posture.

* Lift your hips up about a couple of inches above the ground, working your glute and your core as you go.

* Place your feet together from the elevated position.

* While holding the bridge, pull back your knees and keep your feet in place.

* Gently pull the knees back to the side for one repetition.

* Keeping your hips raised, continue to moving your knees apart and in a synchronized manner.

* Perform 10-12 reps.

Keep the proper posture by pulling your belly button towards your spine while keep your pelvis in a straight line to the floor below. Don't the back to an arch.

Rainbow kick

* Begin in the all-fours posture with your core firmly tense, hands directly below your shoulders and knees directly beneath the hips.

wrap the band over your right foot and grasp one end with each hand.

* Extend the left side of your body straight up until your toes are resting in the air. This is the ideal starting point.

* Lift your left leg and then cross it towards the right to form an arch. You will then guide it to the floor until it comes into contact with the floor along the side that is your left leg. As soon as your left leg hits the floor, raise immediately and then reverse the arch to your starting position. This is a complete repetition.

* Perform 8-10 reps for each leg.

It doesn't matter what height you can allow you foot reach,. It's important to do this when it requires you to arch your lower back in order to extend further. Make sure you are engaging your glutes and hamstrings, while releasing the glutes every time you lift your foot.

Abduction

* Loop the band over your knees.

Maintain your core muscles throughout the workout and lower your hips until you reach the level of a half-squat.

If you have your feet set on the floor push your left knee toward the left.

* Return to your starting position and repeat the exercise on the right side for 1 repetition.

* Perform 8-10 repetitions.

Hamstring Exercises

As we mentioned previously the hamstring muscles are located behind your thigh. They are used muscles for squatting, climbing stairs, walking and various other leg-related actions. The roles of the hamstrings include stretching the knee joint, and extensing and rotation of your hip joint. The three main muscles of the hamstring include:

* Biceps Femoris: It's the muscle that is located on the outside of your hamstrings. The main functions of the biceps fascia are stretching your thigh towards the hip, stretching the knee and rotating the lower portion of the leg to another as your knees are bent.

• Semimembranosus: The muscle is the closest to the middle the body. Similar to the biceps femoris and biceps the semimembranosus can also stretch your hips at the hips, and allows you to flex the knee joint. Additionally, it assists your lower leg as well as your hips via medial rotation.

* Semitendinosus: The muscle is situated between the biceps fimoris and semimembranous. Hamstrings perform the same function as the semimembranosus.

Here are some hamstring exercises using the help of a resistance band:

Single leg stands

Place your band just above your knees.

Take the bench or chair and sit down on the bench and bend your knees until you reach an angle of right. Then, slowly move your body towards the front, bringing your chest directly in front of your hips.

* Your right foot should be lifted approximately 1 inch off of the ground.

* With the left leg resting firmly on the floor, sit with your right foot until it's fully stretched.

* Slowly return to your starting position in order for 1 repetition.

Make sure that your knees are wide at the hips throughout the entire workout.

Seated extended leg with banded banded

Choose an appropriate chair or bench and tie the band around your leg's base or at a level that is able to wrap the ankle.

* Sit down on the chair or bench and bend your knees until you reach an angle that is right.

* Keep your core engaged, stretch your left foot until you feel the tension.

* Slowly return to the position you started from.

Perform 10-12 repetitions for each leg

Step out of the banded step

• Stand tall with your feet approximately the same size as your hips. move your hips back into a half-squat.

* Wrap this band over your ankles, and then place your hands on the hips or directly in front of your chest.

* Take a step out to your left and return.

* Do between 10-12 repetitions, both on the sides.

* Complete 3 sets.

Leg curls lying on the floor

* Tie this band over your ankles, and then lay on the floor, face down with your toes pointing towards the floor.

* Bending your knee, then raise your left leg to an angle of about.

You should hold the position for about 2 minutes before gradually returning the foot back to the initial position.

* Do 10-12 reps for each leg.

Leg extension for lying

* Lay face-up in the ground.

Then bend your leg in order to raise it towards your chest.

* Wrap one end of the loop around the left of your feet. Then, grab one of the handles in each hand.

* While the right leg is bent or stretched out on the floor bent, gently push the left leg until it is at an angle of 45 °.

Retract your legs slowly back to the original position.

* Do at least 10-12 reps each on the legs.

Incline glute bridge

Place the band just in front of your knees.

* Lay on your back, and put your feet on a bench or chair.

* Pull your glutes tight and then turn your pelvis to the center.

Then, push your hips upwards while allowing your knees to open as far as your body will allow inhale, and exhale.

Keep the position for two minutes, pressing your hand against the band while squeezing your butt.

Begin slowly lowering you body, until the lower part touches the floor. Repeat.

* Perform 8-10 repetitions.

The banded hip thruster

Place the band just in front of your knees.

* Sit in the ground with knees bent and your shoulders resting on a chair or bench. Make sure that your heels are set on the floor.

* Press your glutes to the side and tilt your pelvis towards your center.

* Raise your hips and bend your knees in front of the band. Go as far as your ability level permits and exhale.

* Push your finger against the band, and hold your position for 2 seconds.

Then slowly lower your body until your butt is in contact with the floor. Repeat.

Standing rear leg lifts

• Stand tall with the band wrapped around your lower calves.

Press your hands against something solid, like an object, in order to keep your balance.

* Move your right leg in front of the other leg as much as is possible and tighten your glutes.

• Slowly bring your foot towards the starting position.

* Perform 10 reps for each leg.

Hamstrings walk out

• Lie on your back, face up with the band tied over your thighs, just over your knees.

You can bend your knees and place your feet flat on the floor and lift your hips upwards to bring your shoulders and knees in line.

While keeping your hips fixated, move several inches forward using your right foot, followed by the left.

Repeat the motion until you've got your legs stretched out. Then slowly reverse your movements in order to return to the beginning position. It's a total of one repetition.

The quadriceps (quads) Workouts

Quadriceps femoris, sometimes referred to as quads, form the upper part of your thighs. These are the most powerful and largest muscle groups within your body. These muscles are vital to stabilize the kneecap (patella) and also for extending the knee.

The four quadriceps muscles that are the most important are:

* Rectus Femoris: This muscle partially covers your three great muscles. It is the sole quad muscle that connects the hip joint and knee. It also is involved in stretching the hip joint.

*Vastus lateralis The great muscle runs all along the thigh's outer part. It is attached to the patella and femur.

* Vastus intermedius: As the name implies it is located between the vastus medialis and the vastus medialis. It is higher than the rest of the quad muscles.

*Vastus medialis The muscle is designed like a teardrop. It is located on the inside of your thigh. It connects the kneecap with the femur.

Exercises for quads banded by bands comprise:

Duck walk (glutes as well as quads)

The band should be secured around your thighs, just above your knees. Stand with your legs hip-width apart.

* Lower your body into a deep squat.

* While maintaining the squat and pressing the glutes to squeeze them, utilize your left leg to move towards the right.

* Continue to follow your left leg until you get back to your squat position. This is 1 rep of competition.

* Continue to take 10 steps before switching to the opposite side.

Extensions of Runner's

Place your face on the floor. put the band over the middle of to your soles.

* Lift your feet off the floor, and then move your knees and hips in a straight line. Your shins should be in line with the roof.

Keep your the tension of your band by making sure your knees and feet are separated by a hip. When you have your left foot (anchor leg) held securely in place, and you are engaged in your core, stretch your leg, pressing your leg against the band.

* Slowly return to your starting position for one repetition.

The band should be kept from sliding off by extensing the left side of your foot.

* The aim here is to ensure that an anchor foot (left foot) steady while it withstands an extension leg's tension and the band cause.

• Do between 12 and 15 reps for both legs and alternate sides every rep.

Lunge back lifts

* Place your right foot ahead of the left and bend both knees to perform a lunge. Make sure that both legs bend to a straight angle and your right foot lines up with your left knee.

* While keeping your chest in and lowering your body, shift your weight onto the right leg, while you lift your left leg to the side to the side behind you.

* Bring your left leg back to the position you started from.

* Repeat 8-10 reps per leg, taking a 15 second break between reps.

Curtsy taps

* Place your feet slightly larger than shoulder width.

* Place your left foot in front of your right and bend at your knees to do a long curtsy lunge.

* Create the most resistance you can to straighten your legs while tapping your left foot towards the left side.

* Return your left foot to its starting position, and then repeat.

Do 8-10 reps for each leg, with an interval of 15 seconds in between.

Glute Bridge Tiptoe Walk

Wrap the band around your thighs, just in front of your knees.

* Lay face-up on the floor, with your feet on the floor, your hips apart, knees bent.

With your glutes tucked in with heels pressing into the ground, as well as your your core engaged, pull your hips to the point that your shoulders and knees are in alignment.

* While keeping your hips elevated in this position and using the left leg to move towards the bum leaving you to be able to balance on your feet. Repeat this with the right foot.

Reverse back into the beginning point by reverse the motion. This is 1 rep.

* Repeat for 8-10 reps

Bridge with single leg

* Sit on the floor, face down, with your knees shoulder-width away and bent.

If you are able to do this, with your palms down and your arms at your sides.

You can flex your left foot while you lift your right leg as high as you are able to reach.

* While your glutes are engaged and your upper back fixated to the floor, use your left heel and lift up your hips till your knees, shoulders and hips are in line.

* By squeezing your glutes Hold this position for a moment before returning to your starting position.

* Perform 8-10 reps for each side.

Walking lunges

• Stand tall, with your feet spread shoulder-width apart.

Place both hands over your hips at your sides or clasp your hands in front of you.

Step in the direction of your left foot and shift the weight of your foot to your heel. Bend your left knee to 90 degrees. This will also allow your right knee at exactly the same degree. Maintain the position for one second.

* Without changing the posture of your left leg make a step forward with your right foot, and repeat the same motion.

* Once your right foot is straight to your floor, in the classic lunge position, stop for an additional second.

* Keep "walking" while changing legs and lunging.

Chapter 11: Exercises For Cardio

The following exercises are sure to get your heart pumping and are perfect for cardio

Jacks with Banded Jumping

The band should be wrapped just above your knees.

* Stand tall with your arms by your sides, and keep your feet in a row.

* Bend your knees slightly.

* Jump, making sure you stretch your legs slightly larger than the shoulder width. then raise your arms over your head, while keeping your arms straight.

When your feet reach the ground, instantly jump to get back to the original position.

* Continue jumping into and out for 30 to 45 seconds.

*Clap your hands over the top then tap both sides after you lower them to make sure you have a full range of movement.

Butt kicks

* With your feet about hip width apart, put the band below the calves.

* By bending on your right knee pull your left foot in front of you until it gently touches the glutes. It's okay if you can't reach your bottom; only do as much as is possible.

Then lower your feet to the floor and then change to the left foot, bouncing at a slight angle when you repeat the motion.

* Switch legs as fast as you are able for 30 to 45 minutes.

High knees

* Keep your feet up with the band around your thighs, or below your feet, and keep your feet spread hip-width apart.

* Lift your left leg, keeping your knee bent to the belly button.

You can lower your feet to the ground , then switch to the left leg, repeating the move. You can jump up or down when you switch legs or you can not.

* Keep switching legs in the fastest speed you can for 30 to 45 minutes.

As you increase your fitness and endurance, consider raising your knees or adding a dumbbell to the exercise.

Squat until heel is raised.

Stand tall and keep your feet about the same width as your hips.

Bend your knees at an angle that is right, while improving your posture by keeping the back straight.

* Pull your body back upwards until you have straight legs. lift yourself up using your body weight to press onto the heels of your feet.

Hold the position for about 1-2 seconds before you lower your heels to the ground.

* Perform 12-15 reps.

Step-up of the calf with explosive force

Standing tall, keep your back straight and place one foot on the lower step of the staircase or an imposing box that is in front of you.

* By bracing your core muscles and then bursting upwards, you can do the air by pressing on the lifted foot and switching your feet's position.

* Do 15 reps.

Seal Jump

* Stand tall, with the band swung over your legs, with arms by your sides, and your feet close.

With your knees slightly bent, make the legs by a little more than shoulder width and then lift your arms towards the sides, and in line with the ground beneath the level below.

* Jump a second time and bring both feet in line while clapping your hands to the side of your body.

* Keep jumping as quick that you are able for 30 to 45 minutes.

If you're up to the challenge, test to jump with your heels upwards and shifting your weight towards the heels to help engage your calves better.

Forward Lunge

* Make sure you are standing with an upright back and with your legs about the length of your hips.

* Then move forward using your left leg and make sure you move your weight to ensure that you are landing on the floor using your heels.

Begin to lower your hips so that you have your left leg in line with the floor, and your right knee is bent at 90 degrees. Try tap your right knee to the floor in accordance with the level of fitness you have.

Pressing the left foot, get back up, then return to your starting position.

Repeat the motion by using your left leg until you have completed 1 repetition.

Do 10-12 repetitions.

Squats

Stand tall with shoulders-width distance between your legs. an elastic band around your thighs just above your knees.

* Place your hands behind yourself or your hips, with your toes slightly pointed towards the outside.

Then bend your knees in a bent position and gently push your hips back like you are sitting.

Begin to lower yourself until the thighs of your lower body and floor are level.

If your knees are bent at an angle of right and your knees bent at a right angle, hold the position for two to three seconds.

* Gently return to your original position.

* Perform 10-12 reps.

The concentric movement of rising will determine the results you get from squatting. Therefore, sit up slowly and squeeze the glutes.

Standing Leg Taps Sides

* While standing shoulder width, wrap your resistance band around your ankles.

* Pull your core backwards as you bend the knees in order to let your bum out. This is the starting point.

* Make tension on the band by tapping your left foot to on the side to your left.

* Return to your beginning position, and then repeat the motion with your left foot.

Do 10-12 reps per leg.

A Banded Lateral Step to get out of squat

* The band should be looped below your knees, with your feet directly below your hips and then clasp your hands behind your chest.

* Take a big step to the left using the left side of your foot.

• Bend knees, bend them and pull your hips back while lowering your body until your knees are in line with the ground beneath you.

* By pressing your weight onto your heels and then focusing on the glutes, then return to your starting position. It's a total of 1 rep.

Do 10-12 reps and then change sides to the left.

Chapter 12: Exercises For Core

For resistance band exercises you can choose to use flexible, open-ended or flat bands that have handles. Every exercise should be completed on a mat or on a floor that is comfortable. The more strenuous exercise shouldn't be performed each day since the body requires time to recuperate. Rehydrate and drink plenty of water in after each workout. It is also possible to exercise without weights or resistance bands in the event that it is necessary at starting your exercise journey.

Resistance Band Crunch

* Lay on your back and keep your feet at 90 degree angle. Bend your knees slightly.

* Wrap the band around your foot and hold it in both hands, making sure that the band isn't squeezed too tightly.

Use your core muscles to raise your torso and head upwards and then move your hands along the resistance band however, without pulling the band. This movement is made using your core. The movement is stabilized by using the band.

111

Slowly return to your starting position and move your hands down on the bands of resistance.

Each move must be at least halfway between your feet as well as your legs. If you're unable to climb to this point at first begin with the things you can accomplish and gradually progress to it.

* Repetition the crunch upwards and downwards 8 times.

The addition of a resistance band to your core workout will burn more calories than traditional crunches.

Resistance Leg Flex

Like earlier exercises, for the first time lay on your back with your legs bent at 90 degrees. Knees slightly bent.

* Wrap the band of resistance around your feet, and then hold the ends in your hands. Do not pull it too tight.

* With no change to the length of your legs drop the legs to 45 degrees, then stretch them out simultaneously to the sides while keeping the resistance band above your feet. Extend your legs

to 45-degree angles slowlyand bring them back in.

Start with three set of 6-8 repetitions taking a break between every set. When you're ready to do so, raise the number of reps and make use of a more powerful resistance band.

Modification Option

After you've built up enough core strength, you can do the same exercise, only this time lower your legs even further toward the ground. In essence, the higher you lower your legs, the more you will be working your core.

* Your thighs' outer edges, hips and glutes perform better in lower legs.

To avoid unnecessary strain Be aware of your back when you do this exercise. Your frontal core muscles are performing the majority of the work.

The Braced Core Leg Extension

* When lying on your back with your legs up and your knees bent, place the band of resistance over your feet, and then hold the ends in both hands.

* Your shoulders and your head should be lifted just a little from the floor using your core.

* Push your feet forward by extensing your knees from 90 degrees to straight, then bringing them back toward your body. Your back should be on the ground and your shoulders and head should be raised.

Use controlled, slow moves that are controlled and slow. You can gauge the amount of resistance you are experiencing by pulling back the band of resistance while extending your knees. Make sure you keep it in place... It is important to hold it tight. do not want to throw it across the room , like the giant elastic band!

* Perform 8 reps, then rest , and repeat until you have completed 3 sets.

Cycling Pedaling

* With the band of resistance placed over your feet, as in the previous exercise move your legs as if were riding an invisible bicycle.

* Make sure your legs are at the same level throughout the exercise.

* Repeat this exercise for three separate sets of 10 seconds in a break of a few seconds between each set. You can increase the duration as you get stronger.

* You may also intensify this exercise by decreasing the knees' angle.

The Resistance Band's Side Plank

This workout not only targets the core muscles, specifically the ablique muscles, but your chest, arms, and shoulders as well.

* Get into the posture that is shown in the image above and cross your legs to ensure that your feet are over one another. Place your elbow on the floor with your hand to the side.

Imagine that your body is a straight, solid piece of timber. When you hold the plank in place during the exercise, ensure that you're holding it straight and do not allow your body's mid-section to fall... Your back will not be grateful in the event that you do!

* Grab the other end of the band with the hand that is lying on the floor. With the other hand, grasp the band in a place that you like. The tighter

you hold your band better you'll be working the muscles for your next move.

* Pull the band of resistance upwards using your upper hand until it's fully extended while keeping the rigid plank place.

* Slowly return to your starting point.

* Repeat until you have an total of 8.

• Switch over to the other part and continue.

Modification Option

You can perform the same workout without the band of resistance. Keep the side plank in place for 30 seconds either side, or for until you're in a position to do so.

Make sure you stretch out after performing this exercise. It targets a variety of muscles simultaneously. It can be started with fewer repetitions, if you want to, since this exercise is not difficult to master!

Modified Superman

* Sit on your stomach and in the Superman position, with the resistance band stretched out in the front of you.

* Lift your arms slightly off the floor and pull them forward in order to extend the elastic even more. While doing this motion you lift your feet off of the ground just a little.

Stretch your legs, core and back muscles as you are in this position for about a couple of seconds (as as long as you can for each repetition) and then lower to place your legs and arms in the flooring.

Repeat this eight times or as numerous times as you're in a position to.

Back Exercises

Lat Pulldowns with Door Anchors At The Highest

Set-up - A workout is designed to work your back muscles. Pick a suitable resistance band that is appropriate for your fitness level and either place the door anchor on the uppermost point of the door or connect the band to an anchor that is stable above the head height. It is possible to attach stirrups like in the image or simply hold each end of the band with your fists.

Start position - Grab the stirrups, or the end of the band until your palms face toward the front. Place your knees to the level of the flooring. Then, extend your arms until they're over your head, but not when your elbows become locked. Then, you can alter your band's grip if it is difficult to sense any slight tension. Keep your back straight and your abs in a tight position, then focus on the towards the future.

Moving - When you exhale gradually and with control move your fists downwards and bend your elbows forward and downwards. It is also recommended to raise your chest a bit to increase the value of the back muscles that are working. If your fists are only above the shoulder, that is the peak of the exercise and the moment when you breathe in and slowly return to the starting position. It is the end of one rep.

Bent Over Rows with Bands Under Feet

Setting up - A workout designed to target your back muscle. Pick a suitable resistance band to match your current level of fitness Place it on the ground and take it on with both feet, making sure that there are equal lengths on either side for you to work with. It is possible to attach stirrups, or just hold each end of your band with your fists.

Start in a starting position. Grab the stirrups, or the end of the band until your palms face backwards maintain your arms open, but keep your the elbows are slightly bent. Maintain your back straight with your abs firmly engaged and looking towards the front and hold the position for a few seconds before lifting your hips up to slightly lean forward. When you are in this position, modify the grip of your band, if you don't sense any slight tension.

Chapter 13: Resistance Bands

Different types of bands

There are numerous resistance bands available to buy This chapter will provide an understanding of the specific resistance band you might need to purchase and will also provide details on the resistance band(s) you might require. The cost of these bands are still being examined throughout the discussion in this chapter. However, keep in mind that the prices of market bands vary.

At the moment you are reading this book, prices may have changed, but at the very least they will be within the same price as described in this book.

1. It is the Loop Resist Bands

Loop resistance bands, which are often referred to as power resistance band, like other resistance band, is constructed from rubber latex.

They're all-round flat and can be utilized to help reduce body weight during exercises like pulling ups with muscles. The power loop bands are multi-purpose and can be used for any kind of bodybuilding or athletic purposes.

Many gym instructors and gymnasts agree that loop power resistance bands are stronger, more sturdy and are regarded as the most flexible.

This power loop band resistance kit specificationsinclude:

i. Based on research, a reliable working loop resistance band that is conditioned will be able to offer the range of 5lbs to 180lbs of resistance.

ii. A quality loop resistance band has to be well-coordinated, balanced and flexible, stable. It should also have minimal or no adverse impact(s) on joints in the body.

iii. A resistance bands for power can be purchased in a set of three or four bands for around $25-$40. It is also possible to purchase resistance bands at less than between $10 and $15 contingent on the quality, size the manufacturer's price and the reason for use.

2. It is the Tube-Resistance Band.

A tube-like resistance band usually has handles on both ends. They're just like those with loops power, with the exception they are equipped with handles. They are great for muscle building and aid in the quick recovery of knee and muscle discomforts.

They have a minimal impact on joints of the human body (particularly the knees and ankles). Tube resistance bands, as the name suggests is not in similar to the loop resistance band.

Tube resistance bands kit's specifications:

i. The resistance band on the tube in normal operating conditions can give an resistance that ranges from 5lb to 55lb.

ii. They're flexible and comfy type of exercise kit.

3. These are known as the FDS Resistance Bands.

FDS simply means FixtureDisplays. The bands are typically in loops and generally five (5) in an entire set of FDS bands. They include handles. They are sturdy and flexible, and they are made from natural latex. The colors range from blue to green, black, red and yellow.

This FDS resistance band is available in medium, light heavy, heavy and extra-heavy categories of stretch. Its FixtureDisplays resistance bands start at just $30.

4. It's the Mini Hip Circle Resistance Bands:

Mini hip circles resistance band(s) are similar to the power loop resistance bands , except because it is smaller and thinner in dimensions. There are two kinds of mini-bands. They are:

I. the type of fabric

ii. the non-fabric version.

5. Fabric Mini-Hip Circle Resistance Band: Fabric Mini-Hip circle resistance band

The mini-hip band(s) usually feature a cover similar to the an outer surface. It was specifically designed to serve this reason of providing a degree of comfort to the person who handles it and also to prevent the band from rolling in its own time when without being watched.

Many individuals like the mini-hipbands made of fabric since the fabric connected to it creates a beautiful and distinctive. The fabric is available in a variety of colors.

6. These are the Non-Fabric Mini-Hip Resistance Circle Bands.

The main difference between fabric and non-fabric band is the material that was used to make the mini-resistance fabric band, whereas the non-fabric bands don't include a fabric connected to it.

Mini Bands Resistance Bands' specifications:

i. Mini-resistance band(s) the resistance pounds vary between 5lbs and 50lbs.

ii. Mini resistance bands can be reputed to be flexible,

A mini-band of resistance bands is usually classified as follows:

i. The type that is light in weight,

ii. The medium-weight type

iii. The type with the highest weight and

iv. The band of resistance with extra-heavy weights.

One of the most distinctive features of the mini-resistance band include that it's a excellent fitness equipment for strengthening and priming of the body's shape, shoulders, hips and back, as well as helping to an overall muscle stability.

7. They are the Renranring Resistance Bands.

The resistance bands are known for their effective impact on the hips as well as leg exercises. They are extremely elastic and long-lasting. They are constructed from natural latex. Renranring resistance bands are available in pink, red green, blue black, gray, and purple shades. Prices range between $13 and $18.

8. It is the Insonder Resistance Band.

This kit of resistance bands comes in regular, loop and hip band types. They cost between $8 and approximately $35 for the whole set. They're generally non-sexy, highly versatile, robust and durable. They come in five different colors, which include red blue green, yellow, and black. They are made up of four distinct levels of stretches. These include moderate level, light level heavy level, the extra-heavy level.

The bands of resistance in the insonder are known as eco-friendly and are made of natural latex.

9. This is the Light Therapy Resistance Band.

The light therapy bands are known to be long as well as light weight. They could be small occasionally. They can vary in length however, they can be as long between 6 and 7 feet the majority of the time. They are usually not tied with loop knots, whether they are not in use.

They are regarded as an excellent companion for those who want to perform an exercise routine to stay physically healthy.

Bands for resistance exercise that use light therapy are believed to be extremely efficient for women who would like to do some sort of toning in the hip and waist muscles.

Light therapy's resistance band offers the range of resistance from 3lbs to 10lbs. The resistance bands for light therapy is known to be extremely elastic, which is why they can greatly aid in rehabilitation of worn muscles, and aid the process of fast weight loss.

10. It is the Figure 8 Resistance Band:

The band of resistance band(s) are more similar to the tube-shaped resistance band. They are flexible and most well-known for push-ups and pull-ups in a side-ways direction of plains. The Figure 8 resistance bands feature the appearance of a handle at both on the upper and lower sides of the figure. The resistance range is around or within 8lbs to 20lbs per kit. The bands of resistance in figure 8 also assist in losing weight.

11. It's the Lestfit resistance Power Loops

The band comes in various colors, sizes and grades. The Letsfit bands are typically available in a variety of brands with different strengths and weights that range starting from light weight, medium weight, to heavy weight. They offer a wide range of exercises using resistance bands.

In short, they can be multi-purposed. You can buy brand of resistance band from market and online shops. Prices range between $15 to $20 per kit available.

12. It is the Theraband Resistance Therapy Band.

The brands of therapy bands typically have no attractive features. They are typically employed by fitness instructors and professionals as a treatment program for injuries and wounds.

A package of this therapy band could be sold at a price of between $13 up to the most expensive that is available. They're excellent kit for personal workouts as well as exercise. They are an extremely adaptable resistance bands.

The Theraband band of resistance are among the top bands that are recommended by experts for the most price.

13. What's the Whatafit Resistance Therapy Band:

Studies show That the Whatafit Resistance band Therapy brand is/is the best resistance band that come with handles. They usually come with 12 pieces per kit and come with ankle straps as well as an anchor for the door. The handles can be removed since they can offer a resistance therapy value of up to 150lbs. The cost ranges from $15-$60 per kit.

It is important to note that these prices can change from time the. The Whatafit resistance band is the one band with handles.

14. A Peach Therapy Band of Resistance

A peach-shaped therapy band typically comes in a variety of weights, as research shows that they're excellent for waist, hips and legs, shoulders, and toning the arms.

They are usually a resistant and durable band brands. They typically come offered in four different colors. They are available in belt and string styles. The prices vary between $10 and $15 depending on the amount available at the time of purchase.

They are recommended as the best for shoulders and legs.

15. Tribe Resistance Therapy Band Brand: Tribe Resistance Therapy Band Brand:

The type of resistance typically come in a set comprising 5 tubes, 4 loop bands for resistance, one door anchor, colored fabric handles as well as ankle straps. The research shows that they are typically robust and extremely portable.

The cost of this kit may be in the 60 to $65 according to research online. They are widely regarded as the most recommended resistance band kit that can be used for multi-tasking.

16. The SPRI Ultra toner resistance band Figure 8

For the SPRI ultra resistance band designed for figure 8 shapes, a few of its specifications include but not only their being loop-resistant bands that come with handles to provide easy grips on both sides of the flexible latex material. They are typically an individual tube-like item that comes in a variety of sizes and weights that range from light to heavy weights.

As their name suggests they can be used for shaping the legs, shoulders, and hips. They are the best choice for shaping your figure 8.

17. It is the Valeo Long Stretch Therapy Resistance Bands:

These bands of resistance are usually of different colors and lengths. They are typically designed to stretch as well as they could measure between 4-foot up to 4.5ft in length. They are constructed of a tough latex material that has different resistance levels.

One of the most appealing aspects concerning one of the best things about Valeo resistance band is that they are typically light in weight. The research shows that their can range from around between $10 and $20. However, this value is mostly dependent on what's in stocks. It is possible to search for bands on the internet marketplaces. They are a recommended top band therapy brands for stretching exercises.

N.B:

The amount of output from resistance measured in pounds (lb) is mostly dependent on stretch or elongation of the specific resistance band the study suggests.

If you have multiple resistance band simultaneously it is that the force/resistance levels will rise.

18. A Tibed Clip Resistance Band:

This particular type of band is primarily used to exercise your entire body. They have handles, and they offer high resistance levels due to their tube-like appearance derived from a tough latex fabric. They come with handles that are detachable.

19. The Strength and Flexible (Gaiam) resistance band kits.

The resistance bands is renowned to strengthen the bones and shoulder blades and also energizing the posture of the upper back. They are known as a robust, flexible, and a resistant to injury.

They have a multidimensional design (which includes the medium level, light level, and heavy level) and measure approximately 60 inches long. They are available in blue, green, and gray colors.

Their prices range from $12 to $40.

20. The EDX Resistance Band.

It is the EDX resistance band(s) is among those bands of resistance that is employed for working out for physical fitness, and thus increase the mental alertness.

The bands are considered as a great partner for outdoor and indoor resistance exercise. The bands can be flexed, simple to use, and reliable.

an extremely durable set of resistance bands. These EDX resistance bands' prices vary from $9.00 to $12.00 on the shopping online platforms.

21. The Idealux Resistance Band(s).

Idealux Idealux is a kind of resistance band which allows users to alter their posture in a variety of ways when you exercise with it. They can be packed as a kit. They are extremely useful and sturdy resistance bands.

They are Idealux resistance band is thought as being 100% latex produced. If you're an amateur or an experienced expert in exercise bands or general fitness you might want to try an Idealux resistance band(s) for a test run, they are eco-friendly and flexible, making them easy to use.

The cost of the Idealux Resistance Band Kit is between $14.00 up to $35.00 according to the research.

22. It's the 5 Minute Roller Exercise Band.

It is a popular type of band therapy which uses a stretchy band that is connected to roller handles. This is a device for exercise which is designed to improve the overall physical exercise and fitness of your body. It targets the hips, abs and hands, shoulders, back legs, and back.

It is commonly referred to as an exercise roller that takes 5 minutes due to the fact that it takes less than 5 (5) time to complete an exercise using it.

It's good for shaping, toning, slimming fitness, and strengthening. This revoFlex is a great and preferred product that can be used with this type of roller band, as per the reviews of customers.

23. The Super-pump BFR Resistance Band.

This kind of band is primarily used for workouts that target the upper body (biceps shoulders, backs and shoulders). They are extremely flexible, durable, and reliable workout bands for physical fitness. Super-pump resistance bands are user-friendly and simple to use.

The price ranges from $17 to $34 at open markets and in the online shops. They are available in colors black and red, as well as yellow blue, green, and gray.

24. These Ziftex resistance bands.

The set of resistance bands is available in heavy, light as well as extra-heavy weight band kind. They are durable, reliable and effective resistance bands in diverse colours, ranging from blue, red pink, green, yellow and purple, as well as black.

In general, generally speaking, Ziftex resistance bands are naturally latex-based. They are durable, long-lasting flexible and non-sexy. The cost for Ziftex resistance bands is a bit higher. Ziftex resistance band ranges from $30-$32 for a complete set of bands.

25. This is the Physioworx The Resistance Band type.

The resistance band is appreciated for its rehabilitation exercise, strength training and muscle conditioning capabilities. The physioworx band is low in latex and inexpensive in price, when you decide to buy.

The bands of resistance are generally available in seven different resistance levels. Their other features include however, not only the following:

I. Physioworx are known to be extremely adaptable.

ii. The price can vary from PS6 and up PS42.

iii. As previously stated that they're free of latex.

iv. A great feature of the physioworx bands is that , just similar to other bands they're reuseable.

v. They are available in seven different colours and have high resistance tension and various lengths.

vi. The physioworx bands are efficient in both exercises for the upper as well as lower exercises.

They are able to exercise in a limitless way.

Grips

Up Grip

The band is held with the palms with the up-facing fingers completely enclosing the band. It is most commonly used for exercises that require you to row or curl the band toward your body, for example Biceps curls.

Down Grip

In down grip , the band is held in your hands facing downwards, with fingers fully enclosing and securing the band. It is mostly employed for exercises that require pulling off the bands from yourself (with the help of an anchor fixed to the ground) or ones that involve you pulling the band towards your body.

Hammer Grip

In hammer grip , you hold the band with your fist while keeping your palms facing one another.

Open Hand Grip

In open hand grip , the bands are wrapped about hands that are open. It is usually used in pulling the band from your body.

Wrist Alignment

The band must be held in the palm with the wrist in a an upright position i.e. the hand should be aligned with your forearm (neither extended or bent).

Ready Position

Keep your feet straight with your at a hip-width distance with your hips and shoulders set (facing toward the front) with the gluteal (hip) muscles contract the knees are soft, tight thigh muscles, arms to the sides of your body and looking straight ahead.

How to Utilize The Band

Only use the bands in accordance with instructions.

* Do not stretch the band toward the direction of your face or any other parts that are sensitive to the body.

Don't stretch the band at more than 2.5 times its initial length.

* If the desired resistance is not reached When using in accordance with instructions, switch to a band that offers the desired resistance.

* Check for signs of wear and tear prior to use. Remove the product if it is damaged.

You can exercise on hardwood floors, carpeted surfaces or grass.

* Avoid using on surfaces that are abrasive. Abrasive surfaces like asphalt or cement can harm the band.

* Stay away from children.

* Be sure to check the specific directions included with your set of band. The products used for the production could have special properties.

Be sure that when you tie a tension loop bands around the ankles of your feet, you wrap it on your feet using both hands. If you want to remove it be sure to remove it using both hands. Don't kick off or attempt to remove them with your shoes. This could damage the band.

Safety and General Tips for Resistance Bands.

They are generally safer than weight-training equipment at the gym, however, certain precautions should be taken in order to get maximum benefit from the bands. Being cautious can aid in reducing the risk of injuries, and can help you reach your fitness goals more quickly.

Maintain your body in a straight line.

When working out with resistance bands, be careful not to bend over in a way which you aren't able to hold. Make sure you remain in a good alignment while your knees are bent slightly as you work.

Make sure that your hips and shoulders are in alignment and the spine curves naturally.

* Try working out using the bands without them.

The majority of exercises that are performed using resistance bands are standard exercises. Before you start any exercise you've not previously tried make sure you practice it without the band first.

This will allow you to have the knowledge of what the right movements should be performed without straining your muscles too much. It is possible to add resistance bands to your exercise once you are sure that you're confident in the exercise.

* Remember to breathe.

Breathing is crucial and can't be understated. When you tighten your muscles while you are working out make sure you keep breathing with ease.

As you progress in your training for resistance the training will become more challenging and difficult. It is not necessary to keep your breath; instead, breathe out.

* Don't fix your joints.

If you are using too much resistance, it will result in your joints becoming stuck when your band grows. To prevent this from happening, make sure to bend your joints in a slight angle with the point where the resistance band is fully extended.

This will stop you from exaggerating too much and causing injury to your muscles.

* Be patient.

The various bands are colored. Don't be in a rush to advance to the next one, instead you should take your time to master a particular color of the band before moving to the next stage. In general, you must be able to perform three sets of 10 to 15 repetitions before you attempt another band.

* Don't let go of a stretched or tense resistance band.

If a resistance band has been stretched to its maximum release it quickly will cause it to come back to you. This can be painful, it is recommended to wait until you've let go of the tension in the band before letting it go.

* Do not extend the band too far.

While stretching the band be sure to not extend it beyond 2 1/2 times its initial length. If you extend it longer than the capacity of the band the band could break or tear.

Check your band's condition before you put it on.

Before you begin any exercise routine, be sure to inspect your band to ensure there aren't any tears or fraying. In the event of a tear, it could cause an enormous injury during your workouts. You don't wish for your band to fall off when you put pressure on it.

* Keep your band away from storage in humid or sunny areas.

Like every other tool Resistance bands too need to be kept in dry, cool places after use. The bands' handles are to be cleaned after use. If you store it in a moist area could result in the development of bacteria.

Warming Up And Stretches

Like any other exercise that you do, it is best to begin with a short warm-up before moving on to the actual workout. It is important to warm our body sufficiently to sweat and loosen up our muscles in preparation for the exercise. The ideal warm-up regimen is one that involves the movements of every part of the body and should last between 10 and 15 minutes.

Then, why is it necessary to perform warm-ups?

They protect against injury

As your heart rate rises the muscles get warm and stretch, thereby avoiding injuries.

The flow of blood to your muscles

If you warm up the blood flow to your muscles increase because it is a response of the heart to pump out more blood, as the muscle blood vessels grow to allow oxygenated bloodflow to your muscles.

Flexibility increases

The muscles stretch, which reduces the possibility of a pull on your muscles or joint discomfort.

Helps you prepare to work with equipment and machines

The flow of blood in your muscles heats them up which allows them to react more effectively to the challenges of working with equipment and machines.

It helps loosen your joints

When the temperature of your body rises the joints begin to relax, decreasing tension on your tendons and joints during exercise.

Allow your brain to connect with your body

Warm-ups aid in focusing your mind on your body and muscles before training, which improves your coordination and skill throughout the exercise.

Warm-up Exercises

Below are some examples of warm-up exercises:

Neck Stretches

Instructions

1. Standing straight in front of the chair, with your shoulders relaxed.

2. Take a deep breath slowly, and then with a controlled movements, rotate your head to the left as far as you are able.

3. Inhale and then move your neck to the left, then back to the extent you can. Repeat this five times on each side.

4. Return your neck to the original position, and then take a pause.

5. Take a deep breath as you lift your neck upwards as far as you are able to go.

6. Inhale and bring your neck back to its starting point, and then raise your chin towards the chest as low as you can. Maintain your back straight, and shoulders relaxed.

7. Repeat five times on each side.

Shoulder Rolls

Instructions

1. Straighten your legs with your feet hip-width apart , and your arms suspended at your sides.

2. Inhale as you raise your shoulders toward your ears as high as you are able to.

3. Make sure you tighten your shoulder blades as you shift your shoulders back.

4. Inhale and lower the shoulders back to their starting point.

Leg Swings

Instructions

1. Standing upright, next to the chair. Make use of the chair to support.

2. Place your left hand onto the seat's back. Place your right hand on your side.

3. Breathe and move your right leg forward with a kicking motion. As high as you are able while keeping your straight motion without losing your balance.

4. Exhale, and then pull your leg towards you to the extent you can.

5. Ten times repeat.

6. Pause and then swing your left foot.

Waist Loosening

Instructions

1. Keep your feet straight with your feet shoulder-width apart with your arms resting comfortably by your sides.

2. Inhale and slowly turn your pelvis right in the direction you feel comfortable. Then , move toward the left. Your arms should free to move across your back. Don't stop.

3. You should do this for 2 to 3 seconds or so until you is warm up.

Standing Quad Stretch

Instructions

1. Place yourself upright on an armchair and then hold it back using your left hand to provide support.

2. Make sure you bend your right knee and then grab your ankle with your right hand.

3. With a controlled movement move your leg up as high as you can. Be careful not to pull it that high if your knee is hurting.

4. Do this for around 10 seconds and then lower your leg to return to its beginning position.

5. Repeat the exercise using your right leg.

Resistance Band Warm-Up Exercises

Here's a set of simple resistance band exercises you can include into your warm-up routine.

Lateral Raise

To do a lateral raise:

a. Begin by putting your hands on the center of your resistance band, grasp the ends, and then until your arms are at your sides.

b. Close your abdominal muscles and then slowly raise your arms to the side until they're in line with the ground.

c. When you are at the top of the ladder, pause for a couple of seconds and then slowly lower your hands back to the starting point.

D. Repeat ten times

Band Face Pulls

a. Connect your band to the wall mount, the door's anchor or any other sturdy furniture at home. grab its ends with the two bands, making sure that the band is aligned to your body.

b. Retrace a few steps until your arms are extended towards the front and you feel a slight tension in your wristband. Relax and slowly pull your hands toward your face. Make sure that your elbows are in the right direction.

C. The band should be held for a while inhale, then release the band to its original position.

D. Do this 10 times.

Side Bend

a. Standing straight with your feet wide enough to be hip-width apart.

b. As you hold the bands' ends take a deep breath and then slowly lift your arms until they're above your head.

C. Inhale and stretch your body upwards from your hips towards the side, moving between left and right.

d. Do ten repetitions.

It is. Upper Body Warm-Up Exercises

Seated Hamstring Stretches

Hamstrings assist in supporting knees and help prevent accidents, therefore it is important to make sure that they're robust and flexible. By stretching these muscles, you do things like tieing your shoes with lots of ease.

To do a Seated Hamstring Stretch:

a. When sitting in the front of your chair that is sturdy, place your feet in the dirt (shoulder-width to each other) and move your legs so that you are 90 degrees.

B. You can wrap your band of resistance around the right foot's ball and then hold the two ends of your resistance band tightly in each hand.

C. Keep the left knee bent. move your right knee the direction of your body and place your heel upon the ground.

D. Then take a seat and then pull the band so that you have your toes draw back toward you.

e. As you keep the tension in your thigh by slowly leaning your hips up until you notice a stretch in your back thigh.

f. Do the stretch for about 20-30 seconds and return to a sitting posture. If you feel that your knee is strained by the stretch, allow it to bend only a bit.

G. Repeat the exercise for up to five times, and then change legs.

Side Walk

a. With a shorter resistance band, wrap your feet in the tension band, and then wrap the elastic around your legs.

b. Straighten your body with your body's upper part facing toward the front and gently extend your legs.

C. From this point then, make two steps towards the left and then return to the starting point.

D. Continue the practice again, making two steps left. While you are doing the exercise, the band must be in tension.

Deadlift

a. Place your exercise band on the ground and then stand in the middle.

b. With your feet about hip-width apart, grasp the ends of the band with an upright back.

C. Inhale, and then the band is pulled through your hips and knees until you are standing.

D. After that, you'll return to your original position.

It is. Perform 8-10 repetitions.

Breathing while working out

Breathing is an routine, instinctive steps that are necessary to survive, and it can be a bit odd to be reminded of it. However, many people during exercise are not aware of breathing or breathe improperly when they exercise.

Muscles require more oxygen during contraction as opposed to resting, and the only method to get the essential oxygen is to breathe deep and in the correct pattern.

In and Out

The most simple breathing technique involves breathing in during an exaggeration and breathe out when you are extending (Taraniuk 2019).

Let's show that by doing some simple exercises:

"Squat": Inhale deeply as you lower your body to the squatting position (contraction). Breathe out and straighten your legs back to an upright position (extension).

The chest press is a good option. exhale as you pull the bands handles away from your Inhale as you pull your hands back towards your chest.

*Glute Bridge: exhale while lifting your hips off of the floor and take a deep breath when you lower them.

Breathing through the belly

It is more intense than chest breathing and often referred to as diaphragmatic breathing. When you breathe in air by your nasal passage and you feel the belly expanding up, you're breathing through your diaphragm.

Advantages to belly breathing include the reduction the heart's rate as well as blood pressure in addition to boosting the body's ability to endure training (Jewell, 2018,).

An effective method to master breath is to focus on a pattern that involves breathing into for 3 count and exhaling for two (Newhouse 2013). If you can do this as you go about your everyday routines, it'll become effortless once you get into your exercise routine.

Consistency Is Key

If you exercise 3 times per week or five times per week, the importance of consistency is more than the kind of exercise or the quantity of repetitions, in terms of the results that can be measured.

In a recent research conducted by researchers from the University of New South Wales located in the Sydney School of Medical Sciences, the study's lead author Mandy Hagstrom found consistent and regular exercise to be among of the most important factors for an effective resistance training program (Hagstrom and co. 2019,).

Therefore, it is important to establish achievable objectives for yourself. Plan your workouts to be a part of your routine for the month and day. Consider any health issues or physical weakness you might be suffering from. Insane goals can result in unrealistic expectations, that can set you up for failing before you've even started.

Your health and wellbeing are vital to ensure your chances of success by setting goals too high.

Upper Body

Chest

Supine Chest Press

The various types of resistance bands that you can make use of for this workout include:

* Bands of Tube Resistance

*Power (Loop) Resistance Bands

* Resistance Bands for Physical Therapy

Beginning beginner: Use a 48-ounce (1,360 grams or 3 pounds) up to one ounce (2,267 5 lbs / 0.5 gram) bands of resistance.

Advanced: Apply the 160 ounce (4,535 10 lbs / gram) to 300 one ounce (9,071 grams/20 lbs)

Resistance band or more, according to your ability.

Here's how to do it:

1. Place your resistance band behind your back until it's tight. The band should touch your back, just below the shoulder blades. If you're using a loop (loop) resistor, then the loop must appear to be "closed."

2. It's best to lie on your floor during this workout, so make sure you choose the carpeted area or yoga mat. Get down on the floor and lie on your back, with your knees bent, and your feet together.

3. Hold every end of the band with your palms away towards your face. For resistance bands with power (loop) resistance bands you can simply grasp both ends of the band in the palms of your hands (keeping the loop shut) or grasp each end of the band as handles, which is the most secure and comfortable for you.

4. Begin by bending your arms to either side and at a level with your shoulders, and then raise your fists raised.

5. Lift your arms towards the ceiling, then bring them in a tight squeeze on your chest.

6. Return slowly to the position you started from.

7. Repetition 10 to 15 times.

This workout can be done sitting in chairs. While sitting in a chair, put the strap around your lower back just below the shoulders. Start by bending your arms at shoulder level with your fists facing in the direction of your back. Bring your arms towards the front and your palms in a different direction from your body as you pull your arms in a circle while you straighten your arms. Be sure to squeeze your chest while you bring your arms before you.

Standing Incline Press

Tube resistance bands that have handles are the best to perform this workout.

Beginners beginner: Use a 48-ounce (1,360 grams / 3 pounds) up to the equivalent of an 80-ounce (2,267 5 lbs / 165 grams) Resistance band.

Advanced: Apply 160 ounce (4,535 grams / 10 pounds) up to 332 an ounce (9,071 grams/20 lbs) the resistance band. You can go greater depending on your capabilities.

Here's how:

1. Begin standing as if ready to start an upward lunge, but with one foot behind and one foot in the front.

2. Place the resistance band under your back foot and keep the handles with your fists with your palms facing away from your.

3. Begin by placing the arms bent in an "L" shape by your sides, roughly in shoulder height. You can also do this with your hands in the air.

4. Slowly move your arms toward you while straightening them as move. Press your chest with your fingers and bring the arms in a symbiosis with your arms in front of you.

5. Your arms should finish at a slight angle for the best results of this exercise , as when you're reaching out for something from a high shelf. Be careful not to stretch your arms above your head or out to chest level to do this exercise. Try to find a place in between.

6. Easy and quick return to the starting point.

7. Repeat this 10-15 times. It's not easy So don't be scared to start off with fewer repetitions and gradually progress to higher reps!

Resistance Band Push-Ups

The different types of resistance bands that you can make use of for this workout include:

* Tube Bands of Resistance

*Power (Loop) Resistance Bands

This is a bit difficult for those who aren't experienced in doing several repetitions of push-ups every day for the majority of people individuals, we suggest beginning with a 48-ounce (1,360 grams or 3 pounds) up to an 80 ounce (2,267 grams / 5 pounds) bands of resistance.

Here's the procedure:

1. You'll be lying on the floor during this workout and you'll be able to perform full push-ups if are ableto, or you can perform modified push-ups with your knees. If you're kneeling take a walk to a carpeted place or mat.

159

2. Make yourself ready for a push-up posture. Place your resistance band on your back, just below your shoulder blades. place each end in the palms of both hands (under the palms).

3. If you're performing a full push-up, begin with the plank position with your arms stretched over your shoulders. Then, extend the entire body stretching from your back towards your heels, making straight lines.

4. If you're doing a push-up using your knees, keep your arms stretched out under your shoulders. However, instead of keeping your legs straight, they'll be resting on your knees, keeping you back in a straight position.

5. Bring your arms bent to bring your body as close to the ground as you can, while keeping the straight line of your back. Do not lower your hips towards the floor, and don't put your butts up to the sky, as per all the wisdom of any gym instructor that has ever existed.

6. You can push yourself back to your starting point.

7. Start by doing this 5-10 times, if you're new to push-ups. If you think you're capable of doing more, try to increase the number up to 15 or 20!

Shoulders

Lateral Raising Bands Under Feet

Set-up - An exercise targeted at the shoulder muscles in the middle. Pick a suitable resistance band that is appropriate for your fitness level and then either add stirrups to either end, or simply grasp both ends using your fists. Stirrups are suggested to perform this exercise.

Start in the starting position. Place your exercise ball on the floor , and sit on it with both feet, making sure that the feet are close to each other, toes are slightly out and that there are lengths of the exercise band to either side. Lift the stirrups up to ensure that your palms are looking inwards. Your arms should rest at your sides, and your elbows slightly bent. Maintain your back straight with your abs in a straight line, and keep your eyes toward the direction of your vision. Your knees shouldn't be locked. They should be bent slightly, and your quads ought to be in a state of engagement. Your arms should be pulled up until they are parallel to the floor.

Exhale gradually and with control move your arms upwards to just above the point where they are parallel to the floor. This is the highest point of the exercise and is the time to breathe in and slowly return to your original position. It's important to keep in mind that your elbows must remain straight throughout the entire set. One rep is enough. You should feel strengthening your shoulder muscles in the mid-section.

Reverse Flyes

Set-up - A workout targeted at the muscles of the back shoulder. Choose a band of resistance that is suitable to match your current level of fitness. You can choose to use loop bands or make loops by joining the ends of straight bands.

Start in the beginning - Grab the band and place it to the side to ensure that your palms face downwards. Your arms are extended, with some bend in your elbows, and parallel to the floor. Keep your back straight with your abs firmly engaged and looking ahead. Your knees shouldn't be locked. They should be bent slightly, and your quads must be firmly engaged.

Exhalation - When you exhale slowly and controlled, extend your fists towards your sides until they are to the chest. Your elbows must remain in a fixed position and your arms should be straight with respect to the ground throughout your entire movement. This is the highest point of the move and also the moment you exhale, and then slowly return to the starting position. This is the end of one repetition. You should feel strengthening your shoulder muscles in the rear.

Seated Shoulder Press

Set-up - A workout that targets all three head of shoulder muscles. Choose a band of resistance that is suitable that is appropriate for your fitness level and either fix stirrups on either end, or just grip both ends with your fists. Stirrups are suggested for this workout.

Start in a sitting position. Sit on a comfortable bench or chair, and hold the workout band running beneath your glutes. Make sure there are equal lengths of the exercise band on each side. Lift the stirrups up to ensure that your palms are aligned to your chin. Keep your back straight, your abs in a tight position and look towards the future.

Exhalation - As you exhale, slowly but at a controlled pace, lift your arms straight up above your head. Be sure not to lock your elbows. This is the peak of the exercise and the point at which you exhale, then slowly return to your start position. This is the final repetition. You should feel stretching the shoulder muscles.

Arms

Exercises for the arm are crucial as we age. Research has shown that exercises for the arm can reduce osteoporosis risk and improve bone density. Arm exercises can also improve coordination.

Are you ready to start? If so, here are some home-based resistance bands exercises that you can perform to shape your arms.

Band Bicep Curl

a. Start by putting the resistance band underneath your feet. Then, hold tight each handle of your hands.

b. After that, stand straight and ensure that your feet are at a hip width.

C. Next, you should raise your arms and hold onto the band, and bring the band up to your shoulder, with your palm facing upwards.

D. While performing the exercise, you will notice your bicep muscles contracting when you raise the band.

It is. slowly lower the hands back to their starting point by releasing the band , without having your band snap back. Be sure to control the motion of the band when your release.

F. To get the most effective results with bicep curls, perform 2 to 3 sets and perform ten reps each set.

Overhead Arm Raises

As you get older you'll begin to notice you have difficulty reaching objects in high places. But, by doing exercises for your overhead arms it is possible to change this and build your arms stronger and have more flexibility.

How To Do Overhead Arm Raises:

a. While sitting, wrap the other side of the resistance band around your door mount, wall anchor, or any other stationary object that is positioned to the ground.

b. After that, using either one hand or bothhands, grab the opposite side from the band.

C. Bring your arm up at a slow pace above your head, then stop for a few seconds.

D. Inhale, and then slowly let go of the tension from the band. Then, bring your arms back to the starting position.

It is. Repeat this process at minimum ten times, and then do one or two rounds

Band Tricep Extension

Here's How To Perform An For Band Tricep Extension:

a. Stand with one leg slightly staggered ahead of the other, and lean forward a bit.

b. Put the middle of your band, or the other end of the band according to the size of your band and length, underneath you backfoot. This is an essential element to remember when performing this exercise, as you want to ensure that you lift both ends sufficiently to provide a bit of resistance when you are at shoulder height, and lots of resistance when you are at arm's length.

C. After that, grasp the opposite side of the band. If the bands are long enough place the two ends in your hands, breathe in, and then slowly lift the handles up to the top of your head.

D. Stop for a few seconds when you are at the top.

e. Exhale , and gradually reduce your arm until your elbows bent to 90 degrees with both elbows facing toward the floor. Keep your elbows as close as possible to your side. head to keep them in the same position.

F. After that, gently move your hands downwards to press your hands down.

grams. Repeat this process at least 10 times and complete 2 sets.

H. In the event that you had been working with one end of the resistance band do the exercise again using the other hand. Bring your back foot towards the front, then bring the opposite foot to the rear.

Be sure to perform this exercise with something solid, like table or chair to support you so that you don't fall off your balance.

Band Tricep Press

What To Do a Band Tricep Press

a. When you are standing, put the other end of your resistance band underneath your right heel.

B. Take the other portion of your band using your left hand and make sure that the band is stretched so that you can put it behind the right side of your ear.

C. Then slowly raise the band up above your head until your hand is straight.

D. You should hold it for some minutes. Release the band to your ears.

E. Repeat the process using your left heel and left hand.

F. Perform 10-15 repetitions per side.

Lower Body Exercises

Leg Exercises

This chapter is focused on exercises for your legs that you can do when working out using resistance bands advantageous to you. They can be done to not just strengthening your leg muscles , but as well as improving your balance overall.

The majority the exercises created to aid in strengthening the upper leg muscles, however every leg can benefit from resistance bands workouts.

Squats

Squats are workouts that require you bend your knees and legs down, and then return to them. This is the most basic form of exercise, but it is effective if it is managed effectively.

1. Keep your toes slightly towards the exterior of the body. Let the feet disengage from each other.

2. The band is placed behind your back while keeping the ends on top or below your shoulders.

Make sure that the handles are in the same spot through the workout.

3. Keep your back straight and extend your knees in a uniform manner. Be sure to keep the butt out when you do this. Don't use your hands to in the process of bending down.

4. Reverse back to where you started. Press back down onto the heels, making sure that they don't move to the side.

5. This could be done for around 10 reps per set. Try to do three sets, if you can.

The muscles you'll work on will be different depending on the distance between your feet are. If your feet are spread wide apart, then you'll be working on your Hamstrings. If they are close to one another, then you'll focus on the quads.

Lunges

Lunges are a form of exercise where you stretch your legs while you move forward in a direction, then back to your starting point. It can be done using only one leg at the time.

1. Begin by stepping onto the band on one leg while the ends are tucked on your shoulders.

2. Make sure the other leg is in front of the one standing onto the band.

3. Bend the leg and stand on the band until the knee is extending outward. Find a straight angle.

4. The other leg needs to be bent to the point that you knee is and your lower leg are completely flat on the floor. It is also important to be at an angle of right.

5. Make sure your back is straight and firm, then move to the starting position.

Be sure to keep your head and back in the same place for every repetition. Also, ensure that you are using the same amount of sets and reps for each leg.

Kickbacks

The kickback targets the glutes. This workout requires that you be on the ground in order to aid you in getting your movements in order.

1. Make sure you place your hands and knees on the ground while making sure the band is on the

side the feet. They can also be tacked to a surface directly in the front of you.

2. Stretch the leg with the band behind it. Keep it with a smooth line. Then attempt to squeeze the glute in this position.

3. Return the leg to its starting position.

This is another workout that works best by doing the same amount of reps for each leg.

Calf Raises

This exercise is designed to work on the lower leg muscles. Particularly, this exercise works on the calves.

1. Attach your band using an untidy hook close to your feet. This is a good option using an entrance hook.

2. Get your handles out and keep them close to your hips, keeping your hands facing towards the hips.

3. Stretch your calves out as you slowly lift your heels up.

4. The pressure of the band should be felt when you're taking your calves the ground.

5. Retract your steps in a smooth motion.

Be sure your spine and legs are straight to allow the full range of motion in this exercise.

Lying Hamstring Curls

Lying hamstring curls for hamstrings requires you to sit on an area that is soft and move your legs upwards while you bend your knees. This workout will work with your hamstrings.

1. Connect your resistance band around a door anchor using a set of straps that you wear around your ankles.

2. Set your body up to the floor on a pad and keep your back straight.

3. Relax your legs while you move your heels in the buttocks.

4. Relax the calves and they don't make the workout any more difficult to finish. This can also assist you in keeping the straight line as you lift.

5. Keep your hips straight when you lift.

6. Retract your legs after you have completed a lift.

This could take between 10 to 15 reps in one set. Each one should result in you forming a right angle when you lift.

While the last leg workout is able to work both legs simultaneously however, the majority of these exercises for your legs will focus on only an individual leg at stretch. This differs from arm exercises that require both arms. Make sure you prepare your workouts properly so that it is simpler for you to complete an exercise that is effective and evenly focus on all areas in your body.

There aren't many leg-focused exercises that you can do but they'll certainly perform efficiently if you do them correctly. Another way to exercise your legs is to use these on a treadmill.

Health Problems

A variety of acute and chronic conditions are treatable or prevented by regular resistance training.

* Heart Disease

Strength training has been found to aid reduce blood pressure and reduce the strain upon the heart. The chance of a cardiac arrest decreases when your heart is not under too many strains. This can lead to tranquility, which decreases stress levels, which makes your heart's surroundings more stable (Mayo Clinic 2018, 2018).

* Diabetic

Regular exercise can help control insulin, keeping blood sugar levels in check. Researchers have discovered that physical exercise increases the efficiency in APPL1, a protein that plays a crucial part in the absorption of glucose (Upham 2018, 2018).

* Arthritis

Resistance training can help ease joint stiffness and ease pain because the muscles surrounding it are becoming stronger. This leads to an enhanced level of living for people suffering from arthritis (Mayo Clinic 2018.).

* Asthma

The intensity and frequency of asthma attacks could be greatly controlled by regular exercise since lung function and strength increase with strength training (Mayo Clinic 2018).

* Back Pain

The majority of back pain experienced by older adults is due to the weakness of the muscles that support them. Specific exercises for resistance strengthen them while increased flexibility reduces the stress placed on the spine when moving.

* Cancer Recovery

The most debilitating signs cancer patients have to deal with is fatigue, exhaustion and weakness. The gentle and flexible nature of a workout with a resistance band aids in overall recovery and helps boost stamina in line with the physical condition of the individual.

* Dementia

Regular exercise and the resulting higher oxygen levels in blood may improve cognitive performance for those suffering from dementia (Mayo Clinic 2018, 2018).

Chapter 14: Recover

While many of us may wish we could just grit our teeth to go full-on each day of the week and make this journey towards a healthier physique "over by," making time for recuperate and rest is a must.

Our bodies don't react well to constant high-intensity physical strain on the same muscles day in and day out and the reason is due to how our bodies repair themselves following exercise.

When you exercise your muscle fibers are always tearing on the microscopic level. Do not be concerned! This is the reason for post-exercise muscle soreness , and it's entirely normal. The tiny tears muscles suffer from will make your muscles stronger in the future.

It's during the recovery period following exercise, when you're binge-watching shows, sleeping, or becoming an extension of the couch, that you'll notice your muscles grow larger and stronger. If your muscles are damaged it can take them up to 48 hours to stitch back into a stronger state than they were prior to.

Recovery is vital in this process. If you're always doing the same muscle groups every day the muscles are likely to tear , and tear again and tear yet again and eventually break down with no time to heal. This won't help build the stronger muscles you're searching for, and doesn't contribute to an overall healthier lifestyle or body.

We're sure you're thinking. How do I create the same routine if I'm at work one day and then laying around on the other? The answer is quite simple. Cycle your exercise circuits! Resting your muscles does not necessarily mean that you should remain inactive. Train one or two muscles on one day, then on the following day you can work on a different muscle group while the primary muscles is resting.

It's fine to take a day off the off days from your muscle-building workouts. It's still possible to build an effective routine this way. Also, having a day off doesn't require you to slouch around in a slumber doing nothing whatsoever. To stay on top of your daily routine You can engage in a gentle, relaxing activities such as yoga or walking on days when you are "off."

Now, let's look at some crucial tips to help your muscles heal faster no matter if you're on an off day or going through different muscles. They are generally simple practices to implement and require only a few minutes.

Consume your high protein foods immediately following exercise

It has been proved that eating right after exercise is extremely beneficial to your muscles, however, you must take care to eat healthy foods.

For some individuals, this might not be appealing. Food intake prior to exercising and working out in hopes of burning off the calories that you consumed isn't the most effective method and can often cause you to be hungry more quickly and make it harder for you to make it there for your meal, without succumbing to temptations for snacks. In addition, it does not provide you with vital post-workout nutrition they require to repair themselves.

It is generally recommended to eat a high protein diet after exercising, and this is most effective when you eat within the hour of working out. Consider eggs, milk, beans, yogurt, nuts and the lean meats.

It is also important to incorporate certain healthy carbohydrates in your post-workout meals. While protein can help your muscles heal carbohydrates aid in replenishing the energy levels of your body. Choose foods such as apples, bananas or oats, rice or the granola.

Take Some Z's

It's probably one of the easiest ways to assist your body to recover. Everyone sleeps however what we really mean is to ensure that you're getting enough rest. This is at least 6 hours but up to 8 hours of sleep at night. A half-hour to an hour and a half after-school nap is also possible to sprinkle in when you have the chance.

Get a decently regular bedtime. Don't keep up until the early hours of morning, if you can avoid it. Also, put the blue-light emitting phone away for at least an hour before you go to bed to make sure you're getting restful, good sleep. Sleeping well isn't only about the number of hours you sleep but also the quality of sleep, and if you're getting an unrestful sleep due to the late hours of social media it's not doing your body any favors.

Drink Water!

Have you ever heard of this phrase in your lifetime? Most people do not drink enough water. Being well-hydrated is a effective way to aid your body get a quick recovery.

Men need about 3.7 milliliters of water per the course of a single day. Women require about 2.7 milliliters.

If you are having trouble staying on track There are plenty of water bottles and jugs available on the market with measurements on the sides to ensure you consume your entire intake.

Fight Soreness

Muscle soreness is one of the most painful! Sometimes, there's not that you can make to alleviate it if it's very intense. However, there are certain tried and tested ways to alleviate the soreness in the moment and might make it less painful for certain.

Stretch

Stretching is an essential tool to utilize immediately following exercise, and also when muscles are aching the following day.

Find stretches that can be easily done that focus on the muscles you have just worked and make them your cooling down. This will help to loosen and increase blood flow to the muscles. This may not always help remove soreness however it will at minimum reduce it, and often, it can even prevent it entirely.

If you're already feeling sore take a few nice, easy stretches for muscles that are aching and invest your time in these. Breathe deeply while you stretch.

Use Moist Heat

When there's pain of any way, it's tempting to just go straight to the ice. However, ice isn't the best tool for rehabilitating injuries. For muscle soreness of a normal nature moisture can be extremely effective in relaxation and loosening muscles, as well as improving circulation to the area. The moistness component of the heat allows it to reach deep into the muscles, right where you require the most.

Moist heat is a fantastic instrument to use immediately after exercise , and also in the case of delayed onset soreness. Find heat pads that can be transformed to moist heat through spraying water over the surface. There are also damp heat pads that draw moisture from air to generate warm, moist heat. There are also some that can be microwaved, that create moist heat.

Massage the Area

Following your workout If you're able to massage your muscles that you exercised you worked on, do it! The first thing you should do is be a sensation of bliss. Who doesn't want the pleasure of a massage?

If you're not able to access the masseuse skills of a companion or friend for areas that are hard to reach You can purchase foam rollers or a plastic roller to help to get a nice massage. A tennis ball is a excellent tool to move around your muscles for a relaxing massage. And it's something we're likely to own. Your dog may not be a fan of it, but they're able to play with it.

Accept the Injury and take the time to heal

The soreness of your muscles could be thought to be something that's wrong, however in reality it's not. The muscle fibers are torn and are healing the damage, which is an normal procedure that the body is expected to treat within the first 48 hours.

www.ingramcontent.com/pod-product-compliance
Lightning Source LLC
Chambersburg PA
CBHW060331030426
42336CB00011B/1290

* 9 7 8 1 7 7 4 8 5 9 0 9 4 *